Titles in the *Contemporary Nursing Series*

Nursing in Community Health Settings
Psychotherapeutic Nursing Practice
Dying and Grief: Nursing Interventions
Nursing in Neurological Disorders
Nursing of Children and Adolescents
Advances in Cardiovascular Nursing
The Nursing Process in Practice
Nursing and the Aging Patient
The Expanded Role of The Nurse
Nursing and The Cancer Patient
Human Sexuality: Nursing Implications
Maternal and Newborn Care: Nursing Interventions
Nursing in Respiratory Diseases, 2nd edition
The Nurse in Community Mental Health
Nursing in Cardiovascular Diseases

A compilation of articles selected
and reprinted from the *American Journal
of Nursing, Nursing Outlook, Nursing
Research,* and *MCN The American Journal
of Maternal Child Nursing*

Contemporary Nursing Series

NURSING IN COMMUNITY HEALTH SETTINGS

compiled by
Andrea B. O'Connor, R.N.

The American Journal of Nursing Company
Educational Services Division
New York

ᐟ FOREWORD

This present publication is the eighteenth book in the CONTEMPORARY NURSING SERIES. Launched in 1970 by the Educational Services Division of The American Journal of Nursing Company, the series has covered a wide range of subjects, ranging from such areas as nursing in neurological and cardio-vascular conditions to the broader issues of the expanded role of the nurse and the application of the nursing process to practice.

As readers of the series know, these paperback books are collections of selected articles in a particular subject area, all of the material having originally been published in one of The American Journal of Nursing Company's periodicals: the *American Journal of Nursing, Nursing Outlook, Nursing Research,* and *MCN The American Journal of Maternal Child Nursing.* The selection of articles for inclusion is not random. Rather, the magazines are carefully searched to identify the best and most appropriate material, the articles are subgrouped within each volume for the reader's convenience, and the final product is a compact reference source for nurses who wish to broaden or update their knowledge in a given subject area.

The response to the CONTEMPORARY NURSING SERIES has been both enthusiastic and gratifying. This encourages the Journal Company to believe that, through these books, it is continuing to expand its services to the nursing profession. In so doing, the Company is also accomplishing the goal established for it by its founders in 1900: "to present the most useful facts, the most progressive thought, and the latest news the profession has to offer in the most attractive form that can be secured."—PHILIP E. DAY, R.N., President and Publisher, The American Journal of Nursing Company.

PREFACE

From its inception, the nursing profession has been bringing health care services directly to clients in the community. This tradition of providing nursing care where and when it is needed continues today and, indeed, is flourishing as nurses move into new settings for the delivery of health care and devise novel methods for reaching and serving clients in need. This latest volume in the CONTEMPORARY NURSING SERIES explores community health nursing as it is practiced today.

Nurses in both community and institutional settings should find these articles of interest. Traditional roles and functions are tending to blur as nurses in institutional settings are finding opportunities to bring nursing services to clients in the surrounding community and as nurses in all specialty areas are focusing on prevention of illness and becoming more health- than illness-oriented.

The articles in this volume were selected from material published recently in the Journal Company's periodicals. While the book is by no means comprehensive, it does reflect the scope of community health nursing practice as reported by experts around the country. As in the previous books in the series, the biographies accompanying the articles identify each author's background and position at the time the article was originally written and published.

Contents

SECTION I: **Community Health Nursing: Patterns of Practice, Focus of Care**

Community Health Nursing: A Typology of Practice *1*
  Sarah Ellen Archer
  Ruth P. Fleshman

Community Nurse Practitioners: Another Assessment *13*
  Sarah Ellen Archer

Community Health Nursing—What Is it? *22*
  Carolyn A. Williams

Encouraging Client Self-Discovery *32*
  Carrie Jo Braden
  Joseph L. Price

A Conceptual Model for Preventive Health Behavior *39*
  Nola J. Pinder

SECTION II: **Assessing the Health Needs and Practices of Client Groups**

Community Assessment: An Epidemiological Approach *51*
  Sally E. Ruybal
  Eleanor Bauwens
  Marie-Jose Fasla

Health Needs of the Elderly *59*
  Sister Mary Jeanne Hain
  Shu-Pi C. Chen

Mexican-American Folk Beliefs: How They Affect Health Care *72*
  Irene F. Abril

No Shows: A Problem in Health Care *82*
  Carol J. Lindstrom

Healing Herbs, Gods, and Magic *92*
  Joan L. McKenzie
  Noel J. Chrisman

A Study of Illness Referral in a Spanish-Speaking Community *100*
  Rita L. Allinger

SECTION III: **Nursing in Community Health Agencies**

An Internship in Community Health Nursing *111*
  Norma Ackerman
  Suzanne Baisel

A System to Evaluate Home Health Care Services *117*
  Elizabeth A. Daubert

Peer Review in a Health Department *125*
  Karin J. Johnson
  Mary Ann Zimmerman

A Statewide System of Record Audit *130*
  Grace Lohmann

Health Record Students in a Home Health Agency *136*
  Brooke Branon
  Judith Weilerstein

Community Health Nurses' Preferences for Systems of Protection *141*
  Pat M. Keith
  Mary Castles

SECTION IV: Home Care: An Alternative to Institutionalization

Hospital-Based Home Care 151
    Mildred Horn

Comprehensive Home Care for Earlier Hospital Discharge 153
    Elaine McCarthy

Triage: Coordinated Home Care for the Elderly 163
    Joan L. Quinn

Outreach to Welfare Hotels, the Homebound, the Frail 171
    Philip W. Brickner
    Anne G. Bolger
    Sister Mary T. Boyle
    Sister Teresita Duque
    Patricia Holland
    James F. Janeski
    Arthur Kaufman
    Patricia M. Madden

Respiratory Care at Home 177
    Bobby L. Malkus

Problems Families Face in Home Care 182
    Mary Ann Rose

Family Focus—Transitional Health Care 187
    Katherine F. Shepard
    Louise M. Barsotti

SECTION V: Alternative Settings for Community Health Nursing Practice

Office Nursing in a Problem-Oriented Practice 195
    Jeanette E. Taylor

Improving Health Care for Troubled Youths 202
    Janet Garzone Kosidlak

The Quality of the Work Environment 208
    Mary Louise Brown

Nurse-Managed Tuberculosis Clinic 218
    Lois D. Peterson
    Juanita H. Green

A College Contraceptive Clinic 224
    Susan W. Andrews

Rural Mobile Health Unit 228
    Virginia L. Barker

Camp Nursing: An Opportunity for Independent Practice
in a Miniature Community 231
    Hollis A. Backman
    Nancy J. Packard
    Ann C. Reiner

Nursing by Telephone 238
    Donna Murphy
    Eleanor Dineen

SECTION VI: **Expanding the Nurse's Role in Community Health Care Delivery**

Primary Care by a Nurse Practitioner in a Rural Clinic 245
    Robert Oseasohn
    Martha Schweback
    Betty Eberle
    Richard A. Reid

The School Nurse Practitioner 255
    Judith Bellaire Igoe

Expanding the Public Health Nurse's Role in Child Care 263
    Margaret O'Brien
    Margery Manly
    Margaret C. Heagarty

The Maternal-Child Nurse Practitioner 272
    Marie Scott Brown
    Carol O'Meara
    Susan Krowley

Section I Community Health Nursing Patterns of Practice, Focus of Care

The changing field of community health nursing is explored in the first three articles in this section. The authors examine the various patterns of practice evident in this specialty, and how both preventive and therapeutic aspects of care can best be incorporated into the services rendered to groups of persons in the community. The remaining articles discuss techniques used in working with clients to promote their increased involvement in seeking health care and to stimulate behaviors which will help to prevent health problems.

From *Nursing Outlook* 23:358-364, June 1975. Copyright © 1975. AJN Co.

Community Health Nursing: A Typology of Practice

SARAH ELLEN ARCHER • RUTH P. FLESHMAN

What does the community nurse practitioner do that distinguishes her as a specialist? The authors classify her practice into five functional categories.

"What everyone knows and does is no longer a specialty" is an adage particularly applicable to community nursing. In the past, public health nurses were distinguished from other nurses not only because of 'the setting in which they practiced—community versus institution—but also because they had advanced preparation, higher education, and often some form of certification. The special nature of their clinical practice was usually recognized by better working hours, higher pay, and greater status.

In the past two decades, however, nurses in other areas of practice have been moving into the community. Maternity nurses, for example, have found community sites most appropriate for prenatal and post-partum care as well as for services surrounding abortion. Children's services are given in schools, recreation centers, and churches. Psychiatric nurses, like social workers, have moved into client environments to deliver their services. As hospitals focus more on chronic and restorative than on acute care, the illness-oriented nurse specialists are also expanding their community consciousness.

DR. ARCHER *(B.S., Indiana University School of Nursing, Indianapolis: M.P.H., University of Michigan; Dr. P.H., University of California, Berkeley) is assistant professor of community nursing, University of California School of Nursing, San Francisco, and is in independent practice with her co-author,* MS. FLESHMAN, *who is president of Nursing Dynamics Corporation, Mills Valley, Cal. This article is based on a paper presented by the authors at the APHA convention in New Orleans, November 1974.*

Family, maternity, pediatric, and adult nurse practitioners are also practicing in the community. Health care consumers are increasingly seeking a voice in decisions about their health care and, in response to this demand, practitioners in many areas of nursing are recognizing the need for the kind of skills community nurses have long employed. Finally, nurse educators are now integrating community concepts throughout the basic nursing curriculum.

While it is gratifying to have community nursing concepts and skills finally accepted by others for the importance that we have always known they had, such acceptance is not an unmixed blessing. Unless community nurses can differentiate their area of practice and expertise from the area of those adopting an expanded community orientation within their fields, it is possible that community health nursing could be integrated out of existence!

DEFINING THE SPECIALTY

For these reasons, many of us in community nursing have sought ways to continue to define our generalized area of practice as a specialty. The core of our uniqueness, we believe, includes our breadth of knowledge of community processes and our expertise in adapting health promotion and health maintenance activities, as well as therapeutic interventions, to our clients' life styles and environments. We also view the majority of our activities as taking place outside the hospital.

But, as the illness-oriented nurse specialists expand their community consciousness and other nurses prepare to be providers of primary care in nontraditional community services, identity problems become more intense. Compounding the problem is the fact that we are a society of labelers, and the term, "nurse practitioner," which crept into the literature in the early 70s is now applied to community nurses, too[1]. Increasingly, we hear the label community nurse practitioner (CNP), although there is no clear idea of the characteristics of this nurse.

Because we, too, found it difficult to define the role and characteristics of the CNP, we initiated a series of studies of find out how the term CNP was being used by our colleagues in community nursing practice and what activities these nurses were performing. From the start, we assumed that definitions follow, rather than determine, common usage of terms such as community nurse practitioner. One outcome was a tentative typology of community nursing practice.

FINDING A SAMPLE GROUP

First we had to find a group of community nurses who identified themselves as community nurse practitioners. At the annual meeting of the

American Public Health Association in October 1973, therefore, we asked those nurses attending the public health nursing section meeting who identified themselves as CNPs to participate in a later study. Approximately 40 nurses agreed and completed a short questionnaire. Based on the data obtained, we then developed the questionnaire described here. We pretested the instrument with several of our colleagues and mailed it during the summer of 1974.

We had asked our first group of respondents to identify others whom they considered CNPs, in this way we increased our survey group to 111. A few of the nurses whose names had been given reported that they did not feel that they "fit" our study and declined to participate. Eighty-one nurses returned the questionnaires for a response rate of 74 percent. No follow-up mailing to non-respondents was done.

Our methodologies are drawn from grounded theory and field research(2, 3). We have used an inductive approach to our data to find out what's really going on in community nursing. Through the constant comparative method of analysis, each segment of our study generates the next one(4).

COMMUNITY NURSE PRACTITIONER PROFILE

All but one of the 81 respondents are female. They range in age from the early twenties to late fifties, with the largest number in the 30-34 year range. The second largest group—45-49 years of age—may reflect the period in women's lives when personal and environmental changes enable them to seek work that has a new perspective and new challenges. Their length of time in nursing correlates closely with their ages. Of the 62 who indicated the date of their graduation from nursing school, 40 percent have been in nursing for 15 or more years; another quarter, approximately 5 to 9 years; about 20 percent, fewer than 5 years, and 15 percent, between 10 to 14 years.

EDUCATIONAL PREPARATION

Their educational preparation covers the entire continuum. One completed an associate degree program and two graduated from diploma programs. Seventeen (21 percent) have baccalaureate degrees; three of these nurses are enrolled in master's programs. Fifty-six have a master's degree; 57 percent of these are M.S. and 40 percent are M.P.H. degrees. Five respondents have two baccalaureate degrees; two have doctorates, one in public health and one in education; and two others are candidates for doctoral degrees.

Seven baccalaureate-prepared nurses and nine of the master's graduates also report some kind of practitioner certification. Six are family nurse practitioners, and seven are pediatric nurse practitioners or associates. One CNP is certified in cardiac care, school nursing, and family nurse practitioner skills. Other certificates are in intensive care, community mental health, and medical nursing. Several other respondents indicated that they had certification in public health nursing.

When one considers that, nationally, 12 percent of employed nurses hold baccalaureate degrees in nursing and approximately 4 percent have master's degrees or above, this sample of CNPs has a much higher level of educational preparation than do nurses as a whole(5). Historically, this has been generally true of public health nurses, but our respondents exceed even this expectation.

SELECTION OF CNP ROLE

We asked these nurses to rank their top five reasons for selecting the CNP role from 14 alternatives. Table 1 shows these rankings correlated with the respondents' type of educational preparation and the ranking by the total group. Their high ranking of the alternatives "challenge of a new role," "opportunity for self-expression," and "dissatisfaction with the standard nurse role" may suggest the influence of the women's movement upon their decision. Educational preparation had little influence on this ordering of priorities.

At the same time, however, community nursing, as well as nursing as a whole, is caught in a multiple squeeze play(6). New health care disci-

Table 1. Ranking of Reasons for Selecting Community Nurse Practitioner Role Correlated With Respondents' Type of Preparation.

Reasons for Selecting Role	Ranking by All Respondents N=81	Ranking by Type of Preparation*				
		Diploma N=2	Baccalaureate N=17	Master's N=56	Certificate N=16	Doctorate N=2
Challenge of a new role	1	3	2	2	1	3
Opportunity for self expression	2	0	1	1	2	3
Dissatisfaction with current health care system	3	3	3	3	3	2
Dissatisfaction with standard nurse role	4	3	4	4	4	1
Chance to develop clear-cut competencies	5	2	8	5	5	0
Happened to be where opportunity occurred or chance	6	0	6	6	7	0
Other changes in life made it appealing/possible to make change	7	1	7	7	8	0
Need to get out of a rut	8	2	5	8	6	0
Improved financial possibilities	9	4	9	9	11	4
Improved professional status	10	0	8	10	9	4
Dissatisfaction with teaching**	11	0	0	12	0	0
Was advised to follow such a program	12	0	0	11	10	0
Money was available for this rather than some other line of study	13	0	0	13	0	0
Inability to attend medical school	14	0	10	0	12	0

*Number exceeds 81 since certificate holding group is also included in the academic level of preparation tabulation.
**Includes desire to combine research and practice.

plines are evolving at a rapid rate, existing ones are expanding their parameters, snowballing technology makes specialization increasingly essential, and consumers are demanding that nursing meet their expectations. Reactions to these phenomena are at least partially responsible for the dissatisfaction expressed by our respondents with both the health care system and the standard nursing role. This dissatisfaction, coupled with their high level of education, makes their demand for challenge, means of self-expression, and clear-cut competencies fairly predictable findings.

The next cluster of highest ranked reasons include "happened to be where opportunity occurred—backed into it by chance," "other changes in life made it appealing—possible to make added change," and "need to get out of a rut." These reasons suggest that women in our society continue to be handicapped in their ability to seize opportunities, much less create them. Many women tend to be at the mercy of circumstances; this may be especially true of women over forty who are subject to increasing divorce rates, children leaving home, husbands becoming ill or dying, and the general reassessment of women's roles taking place over the last few years in our society.

We then looked at the correlation between CNPs' reasons for selecting their role and their type of preparation. The one associate degree graduate indicated but did not rank her reasons for selecting the CNP role; however, they corresponded with the major reasons others gave. The number of diploma and doctoral prepared respondents is too small to permit generalizations, although the doctoral group indicated more dissatisfaction with nursing and greater concern for financial and professional status than did the other CNPs.

Baccalaureate, masters, and CNPs with certificates show rather consistent agreement—at least in the top four indicators. However, the group with certificates are also tabulated under their type of academic preparation. Master's and certificated CNPs appear more concerned with developing clearcut competencies than are baccalaureate graduates. Master's respondents seem somewhat less motivated to get out of a rut than do other respondents. This may be related to the fact that 40 percent of the CNPs with master's degrees received this preparation within the last five years; the novelty has not worn off yet.

WHO PAYS FOR THEIR SERVICE?

One of the greatest challenges facing professionals in any new role is "Who will pay for their services?" We asked our colleagues to identify their direct and indirect sources of financial support. We defined direct financial support as the agency or firm that issues the pay check. Indirect sources are those funds that finance or reimburse the agency, such as third-party payments, taxes, and grant monies. The wide variety of sources of financial support reported is reassuring.

The largest direct source of our respondents' financial support is a variety of health care agencies: 16 hospitals, 14 health departments, 16 other health agencies, and 13 universities. The latter respondents did not indicate whether their positions were in education or service. Schools of nursing paid 12 respondents, and schools of public health another seven. We, the authors, were the only respondents to list fee-for-service—which we admit is not enough for us to live on. Other single sources of funding included the military, National Health Service Corps, special projects, and a local drug abuse council.

Indirect sources of income proved much harder for people to identify. Twelve did not respond at all; six stated that they had no indirect source, and one said she did not understand the question. Taxes were cited by 13 CNPs; another 12 mentioned general, federal, state, county, or city funds. Twenty-five more designated specific agencies within the Federal government, with the Division of Nursing, DHEW, cited most frequently. Private foundation grants supported 17 CNPs, at least partially. Third-party payments, including Medicare and Medicaid, were an indirect source for 15; however, one pointed out that her services were *not* reimbursable under Titles XVIII and XIX.

How does the CNP spend her time? We asked respondents to indicate the percentage of time they spent in various classifications of work activities. Professional development ranked highest in terms of number of respondents; however, most said they spend less than 10 percent of their time on such activities, which includes attending meetings. Forty-five respondents (55.5 percent) devote 50 or more percent of their time in seeing clients, teaching, or personnel management. One encouraging note is that over 70 percent of the total group indicated that research is at least a small part of their work activities.

A FUNCTIONAL TYPOLOGY

As we analyzed the data, it became increasingly clear that our respondents could be differentiated into several categories on the basis of their work activities and clientele. From this emerged a typology of five functional categories which is presented in Table 2. The groups are formed on the basis of the CNP's primary activity, clientele, focus, decision-making, and the sites in which such practitioners work. Each category is community nursing, plus the specific characteristics of that category's functional focus.

Table 2. Typology of Community Nursing Practice by Characteristics and Functional Category.

Characteristics	Functional Category*				
	Diagnostic Specialty	Primary Care	Population Group	Place or Spatial Unit	Systems
Primary activity	In-depth service restricted to diagnostic category, usually but not always tied to illnesses.	Examination for and detection of abnormalities or deviations. Generally concerned with all body systems.	Wide-range service to designated group: positive health, overt illness, preventive actions.	Concern with widely defined health issues; delivery of comprehensive care.	Management of personnel and resources to provide better health care; indirect services.
Clientele	Individuals or group members who fit disease category; their family members.	Individual-centered. Occasionally mother-child; some total family.	Group and/or members identified by shared characteristics.	All those within the spatial unit; communities, especially geographic; certain institutions.	Health agencies, other health workers, students.
Focus	Problems centered on and related to organizing care around the diagnostic category.	Predominantly on illness as presented.	Range of problems in client groups, especially those particularly related to group membership.	If direct part of health team serving the practice; primary and specialized, preventive, curative, rehab., educative, prn. If semi-direct, work with and through others to deliver care.	Planning with others for care programs; facilitating the work of others to deliver care.
Decision making	Problem-solving processes and client management.	Triage; treat, consult, refer.	Problem identification; matching to resources; transmission of information, and advocacy.	Assessment, client-finding, program planning and implementation.	Planning, assessing, managing, teaching, evaluating, consulting.
Sites	Health agencies, inpatient and outpatients specialty clinics, occasionally specialist MD offices.	HMO-types, OPDs, clinics, MD group offices, neighborhood health centers.	Non-health or multipurpose agencies geared to serve group; school, prison, church, social service agency, outreach programs, OPDs, clinics, urban health centers.	On-site health services; comprehensive health centers.	Non-health agencies: government bodies, schools preparing health workers, health insurance firms, health care agencies at middle and upper management levels.

*Each category includes community nursing plus the specific category.

DIAGNOSTIC SPECIALTY

Community nursing that is oriented toward the management of client care on the basis of specific diagnosis most closely resembles medical practice. Traditional examples are such specialty areas as tuberculosis and other communicable diseases. Today abortion counseling and working with clients with chronic conditions such as diabetes and hypertension are specialty areas in which community nurses work.

The CNP who specializes in working with clients with a shared diagnosis focuses on acquiring the skills and knowledge of that specialty in increasing depths. Association with specialists from other disciplines enables her to develop highly technical skills which, depending on state licensure laws, she may or may not perform independently. As a result, CNPs in this category are most often found in hospital or ambulatory care settings that have a large clientele from which to draw a particular kind of caseload by disease category.

Usually, the CNP becomes involved with clients after the diagnosis is made. She must not only differentiate her role as a nurse from the roles of other specialists also serving the client, but she must also help the client cope with the proliferating number of personnel with whom he must deal.

What the CNP in a diagnostic specialty gains in depth, she loses in breadth. Community nurses, however, tend to be consistent in refusing to ignore client problems which fall outside of strict diagnostic boundaries. Individual practitioners often engage in a number of invisible or sub rosa activities on clients' behalf, even though such services may not be recognized or reimbursed.

PRIMARY CARE

Primary care has become the catch phrase of the moment. Its popularity, as evidenced by the many recent articles about it, may be attributed, at least in part, to medicine's failure to respond to the more common health concerns of the general population. Most people's ailments are minor and unchallenging for many health care personnel; treatment is considered routine and repetitive. Some authorities believe that 80 percent of these complaints do not require a physician's expertise. From the data it appears that many of the respondents with a primary care focus have responded to unmet needs and their own dissatisfaction by developing nursing skills and roles to bring about changes in the present delivery system.

Primary care is generally oriented to individuals, although the mother-child unit may also be served. Care for the family as a unit, generally speaking, is more often a good intention rather than an actuality. Although clients often seek care for a single complaint or concern, community nurses who are rendering primary care tend to incorporate wide-range casefinding as well as preventive measures in their encounters with clients.

Since people are not comprised of isolated systems, primary care practitioners must be prepared to deal with all body systems. The focus is generally on pathology and the detection of abnormal states. The process involved in this care modality is triage or decision making; the outcomes are treatment, consultation, or referral to more specialized services.

Community nurse/primary care practitioners often function at the interface of the community and health care system—that is, in community clinics or at the intake point of larger institutions. In areas lacking physicians and institutions, nurses have long assumed a primary care role with or without the title. Others are joining the ranks of primary care practitioners. By continuing to expand their abilities, this group may be one of the most viable ways to reduce clients' problems in obtaining generalized, routine care.

POPULATION GROUPS

The CNPs in this category—working with populations—provide broad-spectrum services to meet the regular and particular needs of some designated group. Such services include health promotion, disease prevention, giving or obtaining treatment for them when necessary, and rehabilitation. In so doing, the CNP's emphasis is on those issues central to the client population's unique characteristics. For example, experience with counter-culture youth in free clinics has shown that malnutrition, not obesity, is the major dietary problem for that population. On the other hand, a group of elderly clients may well be intensely interested in sex counseling, but not in contraception.

We define population here as any portion of the public which shares some common characteristics, whether self-identified or designated by others. For example, infants form a group, while feminists distinguish themselves from women not yet aware of their womanness. Populations can include those persons sharing ethnic or racial identity, gender, age, or lifestyle characteristics. People who elect to participate in any activity, including seeking health services, are different in some way from those who do not; therefore, the former constitute a population group.

In serving her client population, the CNP may need to organize a custom package of health services by putting together diverse elements of care into new configurations directed specifically to her client group's needs. She may also assume an advocate role for them. San Francisco's VD clinic, for example, presents publicity geared specifically to the language and styles of several subgroups within the city—black, counter-culture, and gay—on the assumption that each group has special needs and a special language for expressing them. Some population groups prefer that health professionals working with them also be members of the population group, since they doubt the ability of outsiders to understand and appreciate their positions and needs.

The population-oriented nurse may be based in agencies that are not primarily concerned with health, such as schools, churches, social service organizations, housing projects, and outreach programs. Others may work in outpatient facilities and generalized health care institutions, serving clients who speak a language other than English, come from a specific age group such as pediatrics or the elderly, or who have other needs such as counseling and referral for members of the gay community.

PLACE OR SPATIAL UNIT

CNPs in this category provide services to the entire range of people living within a geographic area or some other spatial unit. Services are directed to the total group so that everyone on the site or within the agency's jurisdiction has an equal chance of becoming a client. This way of functioning resembles the original focus of generalized public health nursing services, although the actual clientele seldom includes all who live in the designated area. Dealing with the multiple groups within a geographic area requires that the CNP have a broad knowledge of many groups, community resources, and how to collaborate with members of other disciplines.

Examples of working in geographic areas include the traditional district assignment. Others are industrial sites, summer camps, and military posts where nurses are responsible for the entire population within each one. Having responsibilities for a geographic area or an enclave of people such as within an industry means that in addition to concern for the individual, the CNP must also serve the best interests of the entire group. Thus, if a client has a communicable disease, some form of isolation is usually necessary. Such isolation may not be to the client's liking, but for the safety of the group—that is, preventing the spread of the disease—it must be carried out. When the CNP's responsibility is first to the group, and second to individuals in it, then her advocacy function for any one particular individual may be detrimental to all others who work or reside in a place.

THOSE INVOLVED WITH SYSTEMS

CNPs who work with systems have been described as those who make things easier for the rest of us. Like CNPs in the other categories, these nurses are committed to improving health care for clients. Much of their activity involves working with agencies, organizations, governmental bodies, communities, and other practitioners to find ways to provide client services and facilitate meeting client needs. Their work with systems has direct and substantial effects on clients, even though these CNPs are less involved in one-to-one or group relationships with clients than are CNPs in the other categories.

Examples of these CNP functions include supervision and administration in a variety of settings. Because of their commitment to meeting clients' needs, CNPs in these positions make decisions which are qualitatively different from administrators who do not have a health background. Teachers also seek to exert influence on the health care delivery system by working through others—their students. Still others have sought positions in the political arena, some have entered law school, others work in program planning and evaluation at all levels of organization and government.

It is impossible to distinguish from job titles or descriptions alone the specifics of CNP functions as they work with systems. Some would even say that many of this group of CNPs are nurses no longer. Our feeling is that to the extent that CNPs working with systems are involved in advancing the delivery of improved health services to clients, these CNPs are very much involved in nursing.

CLASSIFICATION PROBLEMS

As our respondents defined their activities, the "population" category has the largest number of CNPs, and the "system" is second. "Primary care," "diagnostic specialty," and "place" or geographic categories are almost equal in their distribution of respondents.

There were problems in classifying CNP activities and clientele into these functional categories because of overlap and ambiguity in the way they were reported. For example, we counted CNPs who give primary care to geriatric persons in both the "primary care" and "population" categories. Indeed, many respondents reported activities and clientele which placed them in several of our categories. One person fits all five! She does primary care (primary care) with elderly people (population) in a Parkinson's disease clinic (diagnostic specialty) as well as working in a housing project (place) and teaching nurse practitioner students (system). The generalist lives on!

Ambiguity in the way CNPs described their activities and clientele was not so easily dealt with. Under the population category, we are not sure what "families" and "maternal-child" responses mean. All too often, in our experience, "families" really mean mothers and children. "Generalized geographic area" under the place category is another nebulous response. This is where we put such answers as "community" given by CNPs working in health departments as well as those who report generalized public health nursing. Target areas such as those in Model Cities projects were more clearly in the place category. We are developing the next phase in the study to help us deal with some of these classification problems.

CONCLUSIONS

The data from this study show that CNPs are a diverse group in many ways. Our typology of community nursing practice is a beginning point for describing CNP practice in terms of specialization and generalization. CNPs can be specialists in delivering health care within the general functional categories defined in this initial typology. Indeed, many of us are already doing this. The time for "specialized generalization"—that is, depth of knowledge and skills in such broad areas as populations, primary care, diagnostic groups, places, or systems—may be a means of improving our services.

These functional categories as we have defined them are only preliminary; however, they are a beginning step in seeking to help CNPs cope with the knowledge explosion which is preventing them from being all things to all people in the true generalist sense. At the same time, they can help CNPs to maintain identity within the health care delivery system.

PLANS FOR FUTURE STUDY

We are currently working on the third phase of our study of CNPs and have increased our study group to approximately 200. Some of the things we are looking into in this phase are:

- Where and with whom do CNPs work?
- What is the form of the relationships between CNPs and colleagues in other health disciplines?
- Can other CNPs be included in the functional categories that our typology suggests already exist? If so, what are the characteristics of CNPs in each group?
- What additional functional categories are needed to take the typology further in its ability to describe what is happening in community nursing?

REFERENCES

1. SKROVAN, CLARENCE, AND OTHERS. Community nurse practitioner: an emerging role. *Am. J. Public Health* 64:847-853, Sept. 1974.
2. GLASER, B. G., AND STRAUSS, A. L. *The Discovery of Grounded Theory: Strategies for Qualitative Research.* Chicago, Aldine Publishing Co., 1967.
3. SCHATZMAN, LEONARD, AND STRAUSS, A. L. *Field Research: Strategies for a National Sociology.* Englewood-Cliffs, N.J., Prentice-Hall, 1973.
4. GLASER AND STRAUSS, *op. cit.,* pp. 101-115.
5. AMERICAN NURSES' ASSOCIATION. *Facts About Nursing, 1972-1973.* Kansas City, Mo., The Association, 1974, p. 10.
6. FLESHMAN, R. P. Nurse practitioners in community settings. IN *Community Health Nursing: Patterns and Practice,* ed. by S. E. Archer and R. P. Fleshman. North Scituate, MA, Duxbury Press, 1975, p. 279.
7. Ibid., pp. 277-294.

From *Nursing Outlook* 24:499-503, Aug. 1976. Copyright © 1976. AJN Co.

Community Nurse Practitioners: Another Assessment

SARAH ELLEN ARCHER

A repeat study of community nurse practitioners, based on grounded theory, led to a revised typology of these nurses' activities and characteristics.

Many questions have been raised concerning the definitions, functions, preparation, and legal status of a variety of nurse practitioners. In an effort to find answers to these and other questions about one specific group—community nurse practitioners (CNPs)—a colleague and I began a longitudinal study of nurses who identified themselves as CNPs. The sources of our sample were nurses attending the public health nursing section during three annual American Public Health Association meetings.

Our first report (see preceding article) covered the first two phases of the study and presented a typology of nursing practice based on such characteristics as primary activity, clientele, focus, decision making, and practice sites(1). In addition, there were five functional categories that included diagnostic specialty, primary care, population group, place or spatial unit, and systems, in addition to selected demographic data about the respondents. In this second report, we present a revised and expanded typology of nursing practice.

Following the constant comparison methodology intrinsic to grounded theory, the instrument used for this phase of the study was both gener-

SARAH ELLEN ARCHER, R.N., Dr. P.H., *is assistant professor of community nursing, University of California School of Nursing, San Francisco. She is in independent practie with her colleague, Ruth Fleshman, whose assistance, together with Lannie Adelman's, she wishes to acknowledge in the preparation of this article.*

ated by, and was used to test, data gathered from previous phases(2, 3). New areas of inquiry were also added. Questionnaires were sent to 195 CNPs. After a second mailing, we finally realized a sample of 86 respondents who comprised 44 percent of the total sample. Several had moved and could not be located, some declined to participate, and some were unemployed.

CHARACTERISTICS OF SAMPLE

All respondents were women, except one. They came from all geographic areas of the country, except the mountain states, and were more educated than are nurses as a whole(4). Seventy-one percent had master's degrees, six percent doctorates, and 16 percent baccalaureate degrees. Their ages ranged from the early twenties to early sixties with an average age of 37 years.

Thirty-four respondents held some kind of certification. Twelve were family nurse practitioners, eleven were pediatric nurse practitioners or associates, and two were medical nurse practitioners. Four had certificates in public health nursing and four more reported certification in nurse-midwifery, obstetrics-gynecological nursing, early childhood education, or medical librarian. One CNP held both family and pediatric nurse practitioner certification. Four others had completed independent study courses with physicians but were not certified.

Their nursing experience ranged from two to 36 years; the median length was between 14 and 15 years. All but one had had at least one year of experience before becoming a CNP, with the average length of time being 5.5 years. Two-thirds identified themselves as a CNP after completing some kind of an educational program. We could not determine what factors influenced the other third. An explanation might be that I, for one, date my identity as a CNP from the time I entered independent practice.

PRESENT EMPLOYMENT

Respondents were asked to give the title of the position or positions they held and a brief description of their jobs. Some had combination roles—that is, teaching plus direct service; this includes CNPs who indicated that they either had two or more positions in different roles or that their position involved diverse sets of activities. Administration and supervisory positions were the ones most frequently given and account for 27 percent of all respondents. A total of 56 percent of the respondents indicated that direct client services were at least part of their activities. Direct client service alone was second with 21 percent of the respondents.

A REVISED TYPOLOGY

In presenting the original typology of community nursing practice, we stressed the need for testing the typology we identified and making revisions based on new data obtained in the third phase of the study. To this end, we asked respondents to list their activities as specifically as possible under one of the five functional categories in the original typology. We also asked them to indicate, again as specifically as possible, those activities which did not fit under any of the five functional categories. In this manner, we could test the theoretical adequacy of the typology and look for areas in which our theoretical framework did or did not reflect what is really going on in community nursing practice(5). The data, of course, consist of the respondents' reports. We have made no

FIGURE 1. REVISED TYPOLOGY OF COMMUNITY NURSING PRACTICE BY CHARACTERISTICS AND CLIENT SUBSYSTEMS

Characteristics	Subsystems by Nature of Client Services					
	DIRECT CLIENT SERVICES				SEMI-DIRECT CLIENT SERVICES	INDIRECT CLIENT SERVICES
Functional Category	Community nursing plus diagnostic-disease-medical specialty	Community nursing plus primary care	Community nursing plus population group	Community nursing plus place or spatial unit	Community nursing plus middle management and teaching	Administration and system maintenance
Primary Activity	In-depth services to diagnostic category, usually but not always tied to illnesses.	Physical and psychosocial assessment; follow-up on deviations from norm and health promotion.	Wide-range service to designated group: positive health, overt illness, preventive actions.	Concern with widely defined health issues: delivery of comprehensive care to all in geographic area.	Management of personnel and material resources to facilitate delivery of direct client services	Administration, research planning, system development, maintenance and repair, public relations, lobbying
Clientele	Individuals or group members who fit disease category; their family members	Individual-centered. Occasionally mother/child; some total family	Group and/or members identified by shared characteristics	All those within the spatial unit; communities, especially geographic; institutions.	Health workers on all levels, students on all levels	System: Institution, agency, professional organization, funding agency
Focus	Problem-centered on and related to organizing and delivering care to those in disease category	Treatment and continuity of care for deviations from norm. Health promotion and maintenance.	Range of problems in client group, especially those particularly related to group membership.	Part of health care team serving geographic group; widest range of practice: primary, secondary, and tertiary preventive services	Teaching, facilitating, and supervising others who deliver direct client services.	Administering, planning and evaluating direct and semi-direct client services, resource development and allocation, research
Decision-making	Problem-solving processes client management and teaching.	Sorting at entry point into care system: treat, consult, refer, follow	Problem identification; matching resources to needs; transmission of information; advocacy	Assessment, client-finding, counseling, teaching, referral. Epidemiological investigations and data gathering.	Teaching, consulting, allocating resources, evaluating those who give direct client services	Planning, evaluating, controlling, allocating, forming policy for direct and semi-direct client services
Sites	Health agencies, inpatient and outpatient specialty clinics, occasionally specialist M.D. offices	HMOs, OPDs, clinics, M.D. offices, health centers, health departments, independent practice	Non-health and multi-purpose agencies geared to serve client group: urban health centers, senior center, church, school, social service agencies, outreach programs, OPDs.	Local comprehensive health care centers, health departments, legislative and executive offices in branches of government.	Health service agencies educational institutions in middle management, faculty, and discharge planner positions	Top management positions in service and educational institutions, professional organizations, research groups, management consultant firms

attempt to validate by observing the actualities of their practice, except as it relates to our own practice.

We were unhappy with one of the functional categories, labeled systems, as it did not adequately describe the CNP's scope of services in activities beyond the direct client services, which were also described under the first four functional categories. Because of the kinds of activities our respondents listed under this category and those they listed that did not fit under any of the original functional categories, we deleted the systems category and substituted two new ones in its place—semidirect and indirect client services.

Our revised typology, shown in Figure 1, is based on our belief that the overriding goal of all of nursing practice, including that of the CNP, is to provide quality services to clients—individuals, families, groups, and communities. The objective of the typology is to describe ways CNPs go about meeting this goal. It is not to be viewed as a recipe for how CNPs *should* provide client services. Instead its purpose is to describe what we know from our data and experience about how CNPs *do* provide services.

To reduce the confusion which some of our respondents voiced regarding the typology, we have divided the functional categories which describe the system of CNP practice into three subsystems: direct client services, semi-direct client services, and indirect client services(6).

Figure 2 illustrates the relationship of the subsystems to the client and to each other. The funnel analogy is used to emphasize the system's focus on the client, and the two-way arrows illustrate the interdependence among the subsystems. We believe that the *raison d'être* for community nurse practitioners or any other helping profession is to facilitate the clients' attainment and maintenance of their optimum level of functioning.

Direct client services often involve a personal relationship between CNP and client. These services are delivered, usually on a one-to-one basis, regardless of whether the client is an individual, family, population, or community(7). Direct client services include teaching, assessing, and providing care and managing continuity of client services. If client needs are to be met through the delivery of direct services, these services must be acceptable to the client. To ensure that they are, the individual CNP must have an adequate support system.

No matter how enthusiastic and competent the individual CNP may be, she will be frustrated in her attempts to employ her skills to the greatest advantage without the necessary back-up for the client. The support network illustrated in Figure 2 is made up of semi-direct and indirect client services subsystems. We found that many CNPs function in one or both

FIGURE 2. SUBSYSTEMS OF CLIENT SERVICE

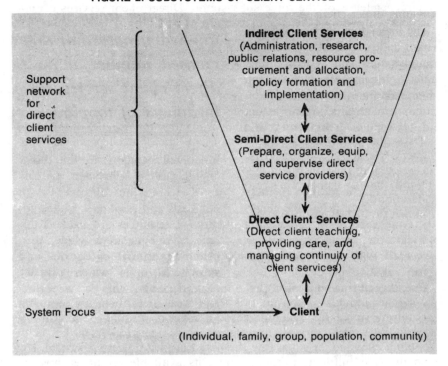

of these support subsystems. CNPs involved in semi-direct client services facilitate others in their delivery of direct client services. Middle managers in both service and education, teachers, and discharge planners are examples of semi-direct client services. The objectives of semi-direct client services are to prepare, organize, equip, and supervise those providing direct client services.

The major foci of the third subsystem, indirect client services, are administration and systems functioning. Incumbents include top administrators in service and education, researchers, management and curriculum consultants, and staff persons in professional organizations, lobbyists, and public relations people. Indirect client service activities, in addition to those reflected in their titles, are generally concerned with generating and allocating resources as well as concerned with inter- and intra-agency functioning.

The majority of our CNP respondents indicate activities in two or all three subsystems of client services. This is another illustration of the interdependence of the three subsystems. Direct client services cannot be delivered without the support system provided by semi-direct and indirect services. Conversely, the main goals of semi-direct and indirect client service subsystems are to facilitate development, delivery, and improvement of direct client services.

Basic to the functioning of any system is the fact that all of its subsystems are interdependent. Since any one system has a relatively fixed amount of total resources available to it, an increase in the amount of resources allocated to one subsystem is made at the expense of the other subsystems within the system. Because of their interdependence, subsystems weakened by reductions of their resources will eventually result in weakening the subsystem whose resources were originally increased. In this time of constricting resources this phenomenon is a vital consideration(8).

For example, the primary care functional category in the direct client service subsystem is currently receiving an increase in emphasis and resources. Unless additional resources are made available to nursing as a whole, then other functional categories and subsystems upon which primary care depends will be weakened and, ultimately, primary care will be weakened since it is part of the interdependent system.

Another trend we have noted is the increasingly top-heavy nature of organizations created by an increased number of positions in semi-direct and indirect client service subsystems. These agencies are in danger of toppling over and/or squashing the direct client services subsystem. If a system is to fulfill its purposes, then its available resources must be allocated so that all of its interdependent subsystems are able to function effectively and efficiently.

CLIENT SERVICES SUBSYSTEMS

The functional categories of diagnostic specialty, primary care, population group, and place or spatial unit are grouped under the direct client services subsystem in Figure 1. In all four, the CNP is the deliverer of services directly to clients, individuals, families, groups, populations, and communities. With the exception of primary care, these categories remain basically as we originally presented them. However, in response to the study data and from colleagues in education, primary care has been changed to include the following: (1) the breadth of primary activity has been increased from screening to total client assessment, follow-up, and health promotion; and (2) the focus has been changed from a disease-orientation to one which includes health promotion, health maintenance, treatment, and responsibility for continuity of care.

Semi-direct client services include teaching, supervising, and managing for the purpose of facilitating students' and staff members' delivery of direct client services. Approximately 70 percent of our respondents list activities classified under this subsystem. Specific examples include: clinic managers, faculty, head nurses, discharge planners, and supervisors. Few respondents list these semi-direct client services as their only function; many indicate activities which are in one or both of the other client services subsystems.

The major functions of indirect client services subsystems are administration and systems maintenance. Approximately 40 percent of our respondents listed activities which we believe are appropriate to this subsystem. Specific examples of indirect client services include: administering a nursing division, administering a school of nursing, working for a professional organization, serving as a lobbyist, being involved in community health planning, and doing research and service evaluations. These activities are all focused on the health care delivery system and have institutions, agencies, and organizations as clients.

Effective and efficient functioning of this subsystem is essential if the other two subsystems are to be able to carry out their responsibilities. Half of our respondents who indicated activities in one of these subsystems also listed activities in the others, which emphasizes the fact that no functional category in any of the subsystems is discrete; all of the boundaries are permeable and the vast majority of our respondents are actively practicing in more than one of these client service subsystems.

COMMENTARY

Several respondents declined to complete the questionnaire because they stated they were not CNPs. Since we know some of them personally, we believe their qualifications, experience, and activities are very similar to those who participated in this study. Some respondents raised questions about the use of the term "practitioner" in community nurse practitioner. It is generally impossible for a term in common usage to conform to a definition devised by any one specialized group. The confusion of terms cannot be *arbitrarily* decided without taking into account the manner in which people who identify with the label, those who use their services, and any others in positions to legitimate the profession actually do use such terms.

Lewis described the debate over nurse practitioners as one between those who believe that the emphasis of many nurse practitioners on substitute kinds of medical skills enhances nurses' abilities to meet client needs and others who believe that these skills detract from nurses' contributions to clients(9). She also states that without further objective data neither side can prove its point. We believe that the debate is less over the effects of adding new tools to nurses' repertoire for working with clients, but rather over the gut-level issue of nurses' rights and responsibilities to acquire and utilize whatever they can to facilitate their work with clients. We wish that all discussions on this topic would focus on ways to improve client services, rather than on territorial battles that continue to be fought among nurses.

We in community nursing learned early in our practice as generalists that eclecticism and diversity are essential if we are to work effectively with clients in their settings and in meeting their goals. From our respondents' descriptions of their functions it is clear that this diversity of practice within the group, as well as among individual practitioners, continues.

Our plea is that we encourage diversity within community nursing practice, as long as this diversity contributes to our aggregate ability to work toward the ultimate goal of helping clients to attain and maintain their optimum level of functioning. We believe that there is room in community nursing for all who are committed to this goal and that the diversity of our practitioners will enhance, rather than detract, from its attainment. Community nursing is a system made up of subsystems that have autonomy but are also interdependent. If those who practice in the various subsystems and functional categories cannot work together in one system called community nursing, then that system will undergo progressive segregation and new systems will be formed. This may be well and good; it may also not be in the best interest of either our clients or of community nursing. We cannot permit ourselves to drive from our ranks those who march to different drummers, provided that their goal is to serve clients' needs. The old cliché "it takes all kinds . . ." was never more applicable than it is for community nursing in the 1970s.

REFERENCES

1. ARCHER, S. E., AND FLESHMAN, R. P. Community health nursing: a typology of practice. *Nurs. Outlook* 23:358-364, June 1975.
2. GLASER, B. G., AND STRAUSS, A. L. *Discovery of Grounded Theory: Strategies for Qualitative Research.* Chicago, Aldine Publishing Co., 1967.
3. SCHATZMAN, LEONARD, AND STRAUSS, A. L. *Field Research: Strategies*

for a Natural Sociology. Englewood-Cliffs, N.J., Prentice-Hall, 1973.
4. AMERICAN NURSES' ASSOCIATION. *Facts About Nursing, 1970-71.* New York, The Association, 1971, p. 10.
5. GLASER AND STRAUSS, *op. cit.*, pp. 101-115.
6. JACOBSON, M. J. An introduction to community nursing. IN *Community Health Nursing: Patterns and Practice*, ed. by S. E. Archer and R. P. Fleshman. North Scituate, Mass., Duxbury Press, 1975, pp. 24-27.
7. SKROVAN, CLARENCE AND OTHERS. Community nurse practitioner: an emerging role. *Am. J. Public Health* 64:847-853, Sept. 1974.
8. ARCHER, S. E. Selected concepts for community nurses. IN *Community Health Nursing: Patterns and Practice*, ed. by S. E. Archer and R. P. Fleshman. North Scituate, Mass., Duxbury Press, 1975, pp. 30-37, 55-58.
9. LEWIS, E. P. Nurse practitioners: the way to go? (editorial) *Nurs. Outlook* 23:147, Mar. 1975.

From *Nursing Outlook* 25:250-254, Apr. 1977. Copyright © 1977. AJN Co.

Community Health Nursing — What Is It?

CAROLYN A. WILLIAMS

There is more to community health nursing than family-oriented care delivered outside the institutional setting; it's a matter of focus on group health problems, present and projected, in contrast to individual, clinically-oriented care.

When we talk about community health nursing today, what do we mean? Many nurses in both education and service seem to be in a conceptual and semantic muddle about the nature of community nursing practice: What it is or should be, whether it constitutes or should constitute a specialty, and—if it is a specialty—how it is distinct from other specialties. Even community health nurses have some trouble with the concept; while there is evidence of renewed interest in increasing the amount and types of personal health services provided by community-based agencies, it is questionable whether such services are being planned, delivered, and assessed in a manner consistent with public health philosophy.

One way, perhaps, to diminish some of this confusion and ambivalence is to look again at those fundamental concepts and approaches that have traditionally been a part of public health practice and note their contemporary relevance. Although such a review may not resolve the dilemma, it may stimulate thinking about skills and approaches to bring about more responsible and effective participation by nurses in decision making related to health care delivery.

At present, there are three key barriers to effective integration of pre-

CAROLYN WILLIAMS, R.N. PH.D., *is associate professor of nursing in the School of Nursing and assistant professor of epidemiology in the School of Public Health, University of North Carolina, Chapel Hill.*

ventive and therapeutic community health services and to the planning, delivery, and evaluation of nursing services that are in touch with community needs, include appropriate consumer participation, and give attention to the natural history of the problems being addressed. Two of the barriers are conceptual ones: first, defining public health nursing practice solely in terms of *where* care takes place and/or whether or not the provider functions in a family-oriented fashion and, second, failing to understand the distinction between the respective foci of clinical nursing and medicine, on the one hand, and public health practice, on the other. The third barrier, in part a legacy of the first two, is an organizational one; paucity of service settings in which the individualistic clinical approach of nursing and medicine and the basic public health strategy of dealing with aggregates are effectively merged and practiced.

WHY SUCH BARRIERS?

Many nurses tend to view care settings other than inpatient hospital units as community settings and to define the nursing care which takes place there as community nursing. Some even consider community nursing so defined as a specialty! Such distinctions are less than helpful, and for several reasons.

First, a very narrow definition of community results when one leaves acute care institutions and meaningful articulation between such institutions and other delivery systems out of the picture. Second, although such distinctions may once have enjoyed some validity, other specialty areas in nursing are now preparing students to consider family factors and to practice in extra-hospital situations. The result is a blurring of specialties and the emergence, particularly in graduate education, of confusion about the focus of community nursing. Finally, and most important, the distinctions cited do not appropriately reflect the essence of public health practice, its relationship to other specialty areas, and its relevance in addressing health-related problems in a rational manner.

Further, in viewing direct care services provided outside of institutional settings as community health practice, those responsible for education and service programs have either completely neglected or seriously de-emphasized the distinction between the foci of clinical nursing and medicine, on the one hand, and public health practice, on the other. *And they are different.* In clinical nursing or medicine the individual patient or family is the unit of care, whereas the central feature of public health practice, according to Sidney Kark is, "... focus on the health of population groups (aggregates) such as ... [those in a defined] community"(1).

Both nursing and medical education focuses primarily on preparing professionals to make decisions at the individual patient level. Students are taught to assess the health status of individuals, to make appropriate decisions regarding the care each patient or client should receive, and to see that such care is provided through their own efforts or those of others. Considerably less attention is given to defining problems and proposing solutions at the group or aggregate level, and the transition to this kind of approach may be difficult.

While the integration of community health concepts into basic nursing programs might have been expected to facilitate such thinking, the teaching has frequently emphasized individualistic approaches as opposed to methods of defining problems and assessing impact at aggregate levels. As a result, the graduates are not familiar with group-level decision making, nor are they explicitly aware of the relationship between decisions made at the aggregate level and those made at the patient-provider encounter level.

DISTINGUISHING AGGREGATES OR GROUPS

Group, as defined here, is not limited to an interacting entity—a sociological term—although in some cases it may be. Rather it refers to an aggregate of individuals who have in common one or more personal or environmental characteristics. Some of these characteristics may mean that a group is at high risk of developing specific health problems: for instance, those with hypertension and thereby at greater risk of developing a stroke or coronary heart disease, or those persons living alone who are discharged from an institution to home and may therefore have a lower potential for dealing with a variety of circumstances. Other characteristics may be positively associated with specific problems—that is, black males have a higher prevalence rate of hypertension than white males.

Aggregates can be determined at many levels. Thus, for certain health-related decisions (Medicare), individuals over 65 years throughout the country can be grouped. Locally, decisions about aggregates are made by community agencies in establishing criteria for admission to service and for the types of services which will be offered.

Such a focus on groups or aggregates, however, is not reflected in movements such as the development of expanded roles for nurses and training programs in family medicine. Instead, these developments represent efforts to strengthen the clinical aspect of *personal* health service programs. While they have often resulted in more available, accessible, and acceptable structures for health care delivery at community health centers, rural satellite clinics, and health maintenance organizations, they have also tended to perpetuate the episodically-oriented, patient demand, provider response approach to health care delivery.

In such situations, patients *select themselves* into the care system, and the provider's role is to deal with what the patients bring to them. No one worries about the relationship between the individual patient's problems and the problems within the community as a whole or within select subpopulations. As the clinical components of these programs are strengthened, individualistic and, less frequently, family-oriented approaches seem to be emphasized to the detriment of a population (aggregate) or community orientation, which would serve to put the clinical services into proper perspective. Although individual or even family-oriented clinical services are necessary for dealing with the personal health service needs of populations, they are not enough!

In 1974, Sheps commented:

It is difficult to find an official or unofficial health agency which is clearly taking on the tasks of monitoring, protecting, and restoring the health of the population; it is not a simple matter to find one that is placing proper emphasis on prevention, and reflects, in its program, the understanding that there are major forces in the way people live that affect their health. These are the problems which public health must address in the future by encompassing the whole area of the environment, patterns of living, and opportunities for the full development of human beings both physically and mentally(2).

Obviously, Sheps was sketching in broad terms a mandate for the entire field of public health, while the focus of nursing is primarily on two of its components—the promotion of health-related behaviors and the provision of personal health services to members of populations or communities. His comments, however, raise several questions: Why is it unusual to see evidence of public health practice? How would a personal health program that is consistent with a public health philosophy differ from one that is not? And, finally, why isn't there more evidence of personal health programming in which clinical and community dimensions have been appropriately merged?

Despite the fact that it is not easy to change or improve the environment, such efforts may be easier to conceptualize at the community level than are personal health service programs. The need, the relevance—indeed, the potential—in personal health service programs for obtaining group-level data—by conducting a community diagnosis, for instance, or monitoring the health status over time of those receiving care in a particular program—appear to be less obvious. Yet, if the concept of public health practice is to have meaning in the area of personal health care services, it must be operationalized in relevant and viable practice terms which are clear to all.

One approach is to develop an epidemiology in practice orientation similar to that described by Kark(3). Such an orientation stresses the need to anticipate and estimate the extent of personal health problems at the community level, without limiting the problem definition to only those subgroups seeking care. Such programs, it is suggested, should have a scientific basis and thus reflect what is known about the natural history of the problems being addressed. Further, such an approach demands a continuing surveillance of the delivery system—the types of services given, to whom, and at what points in the natural history of the problem—just as the status of an individual patient would be monitored. And it also suggests that the relationship between services provided and health status changes, both in those served and in the overall target population, should be assessed.

That it *is* possible to take an aggregate approach with personal health service programs is attested to by the following examples.

Many agencies have difficulty in estimating the relationship between those who need a service and those who are already receiving the service. Unfortunately, most agencies simply accept those who are referred to them, without considering the biases operating in the referral system which may bring to attention only a subset of those in need. Another difficulty lies in obtaining an estimate of the need for prevention or for help in maintaining function, rather than an estimate of the requirements for care after an illness event.

In order to deal with these problems, a county health department in the midwest conducted a community diagnosis as a first step in restructuring its nursing services(4). Through a systematic, rigorous survey of a sample carefully chosen to be representative of community residents 65 years and older, staff were able to document the status of this population in terms of health conditions as reported, physical functioning, social isolation, and accessibility of medical care. On the basis of these diagnostic data, they projected that their services were reaching only about 25 percent of the people in that age group who could potentially profit from them. And because of other data gathered, they were able to estimate where those in greatest need could be found. These data are being used in restructuring and refocusing the nursing program.

POPULATIONS AT RISK

In another county health department, the focus was on a school population(5, 6). The services provided to school children were a responsibility of the department's public health nursing staff. Because of time limitations, however, and with the exceptions of hearing and vision programs, the nurses' school-related responsibilities were frequently limited to one-time episodic encounters with individual children referred by teachers or principals or occasionally self-referred. Response to such service needs may be necessary; however, persisting in these activities would result in an unbalanced program, with insufficient preventive services. Further, children with problems unidentified by the teacher, principal, or themselves often did not come to the attention of the nurse at all. Aware of this fact, the health department decided to continue the usual services provided to the schools while also conducting a pilot program that was preventive in nature and directed to a defined group of children.

How could children with needs or at risk of developing problems be identified? Industrial studies have shown that a small proportion of persons are responsible for the majority of illness in work groups(7). Further, a recent school study indicated that a good predictor of a pupil's future absences is his previous year's absence record(8). The significant point here is that at least 80 percent of school absences have been found to be for health reasons(9, 10). It was therefore decided that identification of children with a high record of absences would be a reasonable way of defining a group who would be at high risk for future episodes of illness and absence and who, as a group, might have more basic health problems than children with a history of low absence. And it was further decided that this was a group to whom nursing services could be profitably directed.

In order to evaluate the services, the design of the program called for a comparison of results in one population to those in a control population. Two groups of high absence children comparable in factors thought to be associated with absence experience were therefore selected. One group received professional nursing services, the control group did not, and the results were documented in terms of change in absence status.

At the beginning of the school year, the nurses assigned to the experimental groups made a family-centered assessment of each high absence pupil as soon as possible. In the process, the nurses were expected to assess and identify possible explanations for the previous year's absence, determine the child's current health status, and assist the family in recognizing and coping with problems or situations which might result in future difficulties.

On completion of the study, it was found that (1) children with high absence records had many needs for preventive and corrective action; (2) the difference in absence experienced between the two groups had meaning both statistically and practically; and (3) while about 99 percent of the 302 children in the experimental group actually received services only 12 or 3.9 percent of the 302 children in the control group ever came to the attention of the nurse. In other words, if one accepts the notion that high absence children are a group with either problems or potential problems, it is interesting that where there was not an explicit attempt to identify such children, only a small proportion came to the attention of the nurse.

Clearly, the preceding examples demonstrate movement toward systematic community health practice in the area of personal health services. In both cases there was a conscious focus on aggregates or subpopulations, which served to direct clinical care services.

An example of the benefits derived from targeting services to a specific group is suggested from data generated in a midwifery project(11). The project, which served the segment of a community who contributed greatly to the community's overall prematurity and infant mortality rates (those who utilized the county hospital in which the program was based), reported important favorable changes in rates for those who delivered at the county hospital. However, a year after termination of the nurse-midwifery services the county neonatal mortality rate showed a dramatic increase to 30.0 (per 1,000 live births) from 17.6 during the last year of the program. This shift in county-level rates suggests that the subpopulation in the county contributing the most to high rates is the subpopulation the program served.

In summary, much more attention needs to be given to the distinction between diagnosis, treatment, and evaluation at the individual patient level (the focus of clinical nursing) and at the aggregate level (the focus of public health). And, after acknowledging the distinction, we need to consider carefully what it means to think in aggregate terms and how clinical and aggregate approaches interrelate.

Such thinking is not only the route to more effective service, which is directed to those most likely to benefit, but it is necessary if we are to implement appropriate priorities for clinical practice. In addition, this type of thinking is necessary for the development and effective use of a knowledge base for practice—that is, the appropriate generation and application of research findings. Finally, such an approach is essential to meaningful collaboration with other disciplines and to the actualization of leadership in health care delivery.

COMMUNITY HEALTH PRACTICE SKILLS

Although a group orientation is an essential feature of public health, other characteristics also distinguish community health practice from clinical orientations. For instance, careful consideration must be given to the health status of *many* aggregates. These aggregates may be defined in various ways—infants during their first year, expectant mothers, children of school age, the older population, or those who have just experienced the death of a spouse. A public health orientation demands attention to multiple and sometimes overlapping aggregates as opposed to concern for only one or two specific subgroups, as in the case of clinical specialties such as midwifery or pediatrics.

Further, if practice is to be consistent with public health philosophy, attention must be given to the influence of environmental factors (physical, biological, and sociocultural) on the health of populations, and priority must be given to preventive and health maintenance strategies over curative strategies.

The skills necessary to deal with aggregates, particularly multiple aggregates, are different from those needed for clinical practice. Although some persons may be prepared to function effectively at both levels, it is questionable how realistic such an expectation could be. In the past, failure to recognize this distinction has led to neglect or merely superficial development of skills for dealing with decision making at the aggregate level. Learning these skills is as demanding and time-consuming as developing advanced clinical skills. Therefore, within service settings, it seems reasonable to have both types of skills represented on the staff. Since it may be impossible to have both types of skills in the same person, then communication and collaboration among the staff should be emphasized.

The examples used in this paper focused on the application of selected analytical and measurement skills in both epidemiology and biostatistics to programming for the delivery of personal health services. However, as the following recommendation on higher education for public health points out, such skills represent only one of several deemed essential for public health practice.

In order to produce professional personnel with the appropriate knowledge, skills, and perspective so that they might deal effectively with the new challenges in public health, all institutions providing higher education for public health should build their educational programs on the unique knowledge base for public health. This combines the three elements central and generic to public health with content from many related fields such as medicine and other patient care disciplines; economics, political science, and sociology; biology and the physical sciences. The elements central to public health are the measurement and analytic sciences of epidemiology and biostatistics; social policy and the history and philosophy of public health; and the principles of management and organization for public health. This knowledge base may be modified and expanded with changes in the nature and scope of health problems and the techniques used to deal with them, but an appropriate mix of its central elements with selected related fields is crucial to the effectiveness of any program of higher education for public health(12).

From a service perspective, it is clear that if nurses are going to have a meaningful role in making policy decisions that deal with aggregates and thus share in determining the boundaries within which direct care providers shall function, nursing educators must give attention to turning out graduates with skill in one of the three areas central to public health practice. Historically, graduate nursing programs in both schools of nursing and of public health have offered programs in nursing administration and nursing supervision. Yet it can be argued that those programs have not given sufficient attention to such matters as policy analysis and development and the use of epidemiology in making practice decisions.

What about the future? Although I did not intend to carve out a specialty area for community health nursing, the potential of approaches long associated with public health practice indicate a need for a broader perspective in the preparation of nurses at the graduate level. In addition to programs to prepare direct care providers such as nurse practitioners, much more attention must be given to the preparation of nurses at the master's and doctoral level whose focus will be on aggregate level decision-making. Although not completely separate, the two types of skills are different.

Further, just as direct care clinicians may concentrate on the care of one type of patient defined in terms of age or problems, those preparing for aggregate decision making may focus on developing one of the variety of skills necessary at that level. In addition, there is a serious need for (1) providing core content in the aggregate level skills for those focusing on preparing for specific clinical roles, and (2) developing practice models which clearly demonstrate effective collaboration between clinical approaches and strategies for dealing with aggregates. This is necessary if nursing is to prepare a cadre of professionals who have not only developed skill in their own areas of decision making but who appreciate the context of their practice and can work in a complementary manner with others.

REFERENCES

1. KARK, SIDNEY. *Epidemiology and Community Medicine.* New York, Appleton-Century-Crofts, 1974, p. 319.
2. SHEPS, C. G. Crisis in schools of public health: the issues. *The Body Politic* (School of Public Health at the University of North Carolina, Chapel Hill) 2:3, Aug. 1974.
3. KARK, *op. cit.*
4. MANAGAN, DOROTHY, AND OTHERS. Older adults: a community survey of health needs. *Nurs. Res.* 23:426-432, Sept.-Oct. 1974.
5. TUTHILL, R. W., AND OTHERS. Evaluating a school health program focused on high absence pupils: a research design. *Am. J. Public Health* 62:40-42, Jan. 1972.
6. LONG, G. V., AND OTHERS. Evaluation of a school health program directed to children with history of high absence: a focus for nursing intervention. *Am. J. Public Health* 65:388-393, Apr. 1975.
7. HINKLE, L. E. JR., AND OTHERS. Continuity of patterns of illness and the prediction of future health. *J. Occup. Med.* 3:417-423, Sept. 1961.
8. ROBERTS, D. E., AND OTHERS. Epidemiological analysis in school populations as a basis for change in school nursing practice. *Am. J. Public Health* 59:2157-2167, Dec. 1969.
9. ROGERS, K. D., AND REESE, GRACE. Health studies—presumably normal high school students; Part 2. Absence from school. *Am. J. Dis. Child* 109:9-27, Jan. 1965.
10. SCHOOL absenteeism. *Stat. Bull.* (Metropolitan Life) 31:4-7, 1950.
11. LEVY, B. S., AND OTHERS. Reducing neonatal mortality rate with nurse-midwives. *Am. J. Obstet. Gynecol.* 109:53, Jan. 1, 1971.
12. MILBANK MEMORIAL FUND *Commission Higher Education for Public Health.* Cecil G. Sheps, chairman. New York, PRODIST, 1976, Recommendation No. 3, pp. 74-75.

From the *American Journal of Nursing* 76:444-446, Mar. 1976. Copyright © 1976. AJN Co.

Encouraging Client Self-Discovery

CARRIE JO BRADEN • JOSEPH L. PRICE

Four facets of community health nursing behavior help clients to develop their self-reliance.

The humanistic psychology of such theorists as Abraham Maslow, Carl Rogers, and Rollo May is affecting nursing practice. Increased awareness of patients' rights to make decisions about their own care is one major effect of self-actualizing theory, and this awareness has hastened the growth of the nurse's patient-advocate role.

Clarifying communications between patients and health care professionals is important, but the advocate role must be more comprehensive. Many patients need help to be more sophisticated planners for their own health care, an ability that does not come naturally to most people. It involves viewing one's self as worthy.

Community health nurses are in a strategic position to promote patient self-discovery. Their case loads often are composed of people who are coping with everyday maturational and situational crises. Such people are basically well but need support in dealing with ordinary stresses. These are the people best able to benefit from self-actualizing theory. They can be helped with the four difficult challenges of *choice, expectations, interaction,* and *personal meaning.*

CHOICE

Community health nurses have a long acquaintance with patients' abil-

CARRIE JO BRADEN, R.N., M.S., *is an assistant professor, Mississippi College School of Nursing, Clinton, Miss. She has been a community health nurse in Canada.* JOSEPH L. PRICE, PH.D., *was a special lecturer in psychiatric nursing, Texas Women's University, Houston Center, Texas Medical Center, and a resident in medical psychology and ethics, Texas Medical Center, when this article was written.*

ity to accept or reject nursing services. Patients in their own homes can choose not to open the door.

If one remembers the element of choice, the home visit can be an opportunity for trying out ideas, testing skills, and using knowledge in varied ways. Only through such means can the patient discover his strengths and limitations and learn how to use his strengths to overcome his limitations.

Making appropriate choices involves putting together difficult and complex skills. The challenge of choice can stimulate growth or it can be overwhelming. What is most important to remember is that even the most immature families or patients must be given starting points for choice making. Otherwise, how will they grow in using judgment?

Any challenge of choice must be offered with faith in the patient's ability to make decisions. It must also be a challenge so geared to judgmental maturity that, once offered, it need not be retracted. Withdrawing choice may convince patients that the nurse has little faith in them and is a fraud.

Consider the following common situation: Ms. S. is the mother of a five-week-old, premature infant, who remained in the hospital for additional care and weight gain. Ms. S. lives with two sisters, each with an infant less than four months old. There are also three other preschool children.

During the nurse's home visits made over three months, she saw several other persons sleeping, eating, and watching television. Subtle questions to learn how they were related to the family were ignored.

The house had broken windows repaired with tape and newspaper, no screens, and insufficient heating. The children were inadequately clothed.

All the adults present disciplined the children, most often with loud commands and threats. All three mothers took the preschoolers and infants to well child clinic regularly and used free clinic services for illness.

Ms. S. remained passive during most nursing visits, but her sister Ms. L. used the nurse as a source of health information. The third sister usually was not present.

Two weeks before the premature infant was to be released from the hospital, Ms. S. said that no further nursing visits would be necessary. The nurse wished to validate the decision with Ms. L., because she had used the nurse's services. Ms. L. agreed with her sister. A change of nurses was offered as an alternative. The answer remained firm—no nurse.

Nurses often react in one of two ways to such rejections. They may denounce families angrily as being unable to accept help (usually around the coffee pot at the health station). Or sometimes the nurse doggedly returns, her frustration mounting over no response to knocks on the door or strangers telling her that those she seeks are out for the day. Neither reaction facilitates the nurse's acceptance of families nor fosters family self-discovery. What then can the nurse do?

Accepting the family's decision is the first step. The nurse's validation with Ms. S.'s sister and her offer to send a different nurse were appropriate short-range interventions. For longer-term considerations, then, the nurse must be able to say, "You've decided not to have a nurse visit and I will honor this decision."

The nurse must also agree that the family may be able to succeed in their decision. "Your baby will need some special care when he comes home, because he was born early and was so small. You'll be able to provide this special care if you can get the correct information on what to look for and what to do. Since you and your sisters have not cared for a premature baby before, I wonder where you will go for the information you need?"

The patient has another opportunity to decide on continued visits in the event that she made the early choice in haste. If she rejects this opportunity, the nurse should reinforce the positive, "You and your sisters have made good use of the well child clinic for all the children. You also know where to go when one of them or you are sick. The new baby is eligible for these same services. I'll tell the clinic nurse about your baby so that when you bring him in she'll understand the things you'll need to know."

Then, the nurse can leave.

Choice must be offered with freedom to make mistakes, remembering that "mistakes" are only labeled as such because of our own biases. Situations that do not permit mistakes limit the patient's freedom and his willingness to choose.

Ms. S. did bring the infant to the well child clinic. After two months, she requested visits by a nurse. During the home visits, Ms. S. said that she had refused visits because she had feared that the nurse would turn her in to the police. One of the unidentified persons the nurse had seen during earlier visits was Ms. S.'s brother, who had been involved in drug traffic.

Being allowed to choose and having the choice accepted made the difference in her ability to trust and to make better decisions for her infant.

EXPECTATIONS

Like everyone else, nurses operate out of cultural perceptual biases. Awareness of these biases helps nurses develop behavioral expectations not limited to culturally based ones.

The most important expectations to consider are related to the quality of behavior. Nurses have had the experience of bringing forth the best from a patient by expecting his best. Nurses who expect the worst get just that.

Each time a nurse arranges an appointment for a patient who can dial a telephone, she demonstrates the expectation that the patient is incapable of doing just that. The following situation is illustrative.

Ms. D., a 28-year-old mother of four preschoolers, has a long history of service from community health nurses, focused on improving the children's health. All exhibit signs of nutritional and emotional neglect. The oldest child has had active tuberculosis and the others are positive reactors.

Several service organizations have been involved with Ms. D., most notably the welfare department. Repeated efforts to remove the children from the home have always broken down when Ms. D. caught wind of the plan and moved out of the city temporarily. She would ask agencies for service when sufficient time had passed to remove the child-neglect threat.

She was capable of keeping clinic appointments and giving the children the appropriate medications. Usually though, Ms. D. soon neglected them.

Ear infections, impetigo, and bronchial infections soon reappeared.

For the most part, nurses assumed a checking-up role with Ms. D., making appointments and transportation arrangements, and counting the pills left in a bottle to determine if Ms. D. was giving them to the children.

Such complicated family situations can be approached positively. The concept of responsible ownership must be clearly understood. No nurse is responsible for a patient's behavior change. Each person is responsible for himself. Change occurs most effectively from the inside out, not the outside in. The rationalization, "But I've always had that problem," is common and is evidence that too many people have insufficient self-expectations. The "but what can I do about it?" apathetic retort suggests depression and defeatism, due in part to lack of positive expectation.

Nurses had assumed ownership of Ms. D.'s mothering role. Their behavior said, "You are not capable of mothering your children. You are not able to do the things that will maintain your children's health. Therefore, I will do these things for you." Ms. D. was bombarded with negative expectations from the professionals who were supposedly there to support her in assuming responsibilities. She was also "set up" with the expectation that she would fail. Sure enough, she did.

A new nurse decided to clarify ownership during the first home visit. "As your community health nurse, I can do the following things. . . ."

When Ms. D. requested services not provided by the nurse, the nurse stated directly, "I cannot provide transportation to clinics," and explored with Ms. D. her ownership responsibility and resources.

You are the mother of these children. They are too young to make their own arrangements to receive health care. It seems to me it's your responsibility to see that they get what they need to be healthy. I can tell you what is available, but you'll have to make the arrangements and carry out the details. How do you take the children to your mother's?

You need something the clinic provides. You have transportation by bus when you wish to visit your mother. The bus also goes to the clinic building.

Visits ended with some such positive expectation as "You can tell me what you found out from the clinic doctor the next time I visit." The nurse also allowed Ms. D. to decide the time of the next home visit.

It would have been unrealistic to expect an immediate change in Ms. D.'s behavior. But one important change was made in the nurse's behavior. She no longer felt guilty if Ms. D. did not make her own clinic appointments. The statement during the next home visit, "You decided not to go to clinic," was sufficient follow-up. True acceptance of patient autonomy is based on this ability to distinguish what a nurse is responsible for from what the patient owns. Ms. D.'s provision of health care for her children did improve.

The challenge of interaction is not limited to that between nurse and patient. The patient needs opportunities to test out newly learned behaviors with others. The immediate family is of first concern. When one member becomes adept at decision making, others in the family are affected. When a woman suddenly gains enough feeling of self-worth to make decisions, her husband may feel threatened by partial loss of a decision-making role. As much as possible, the nurse should intervene with all members.

Among other interaction activities are self-growth groups, which community health nurses lead or refer patients to. These groups may begin with a common need for information—prenatal classes, adolescent diet, and so forth. Parents Anonymous, for example, helps parents who have difficulty relating well to their children.

PERSONAL MEANING

Threatening or temporarily damaging situations can sometimes result in patients' eventual good. However, the community health nurse should be interested in providing patients with experiences that are relevant to their need gratification, background, interests, and physical condition.

Choice, expectations, interaction, and personal meaning may operate simultaneously. Together they represent the acme in opportunity for discovery and development of human potential. The following case summary shows evidence of a client's self-discovery through successfully meeting these four challenges.

Ms. G., aged 31, mother of five boys, faced another unplanned, unwanted pregnancy. Due to poverty, substandard housing, and a hyperactive son, she was inundated with other equally disturbing stresses. At the time of the nurse's initial home visit—made on a school referral concerning the hyperactive child—Ms. G. was immobilized by her situation. She could not even decide what to prepare for the family's dinner. That decision was the first the nurse assisted with.

By supportive refocusing and by the nurse's expectation that Ms. G. could successfully resolve her situation, Ms. G. was able to decide that dealing with this pregnancy and taking action to prevent future pregnancies were her most important needs. She also decided to wait until later to work more directly with her son's hyperactivity. The nurse allowed Ms. G. to establish her own need priority rather than immediately following through with the school's referral.

The tenets of Ms. G.'s faith did not permit birth control. Her mother and sisters adhered to this religious philosophy and strongly opposed any moves she made away from it.

Mr. G., on the other hand, supported Ms. G.'s decision and was able to help considerably, once Ms. G. identified him as a strength she had not relied on since becoming pregnant again. She was able to isolate her feelings of anger toward him and deal directly with these feelings rather than withdrawing. Through these decision-making experiences, Ms. G. discovered in herself strengths she had never recognized.

The nurse had to leave Ms. G. before the baby was due, but, without the support of a nurse, she followed through with having a tubal ligation. To accomplish this, she had to discharge herself from the religious hospital where she had delivered her sixth son, enter a community hospital, and find a new physician. She had to confront her mother and sisters and risk being alienated from them. (They did eventually accept her actions.)

Ms. G. did all of this out of her newly discovered selfhood. The other multiple problems did not disappear from this woman's life, but she was able to assume a more active role in seeking solutions. She also has been active in promoting self-discovery in her husband and children. All of this from a woman who could not at one point in her life decide what to cook for dinner.

Assistance that encourages the growth of patients' autonomy and integrity opposes interference, untimely intervention, premature labeling, lack of involvement, and lack of individualization. Whatever community health goals are sought, their realization depends, in part, on abiding faith in all human-kind's inherent potential for self-actualization.

From *Nursing Outlook* 23:385-390, June 1975. Copyright © 1975. AJN Co.

A Conceptual Model for Preventive Health Behavior

NOLA J. PENDER

Personal, interpersonal, and situational factors are the motivating or inhibiting determinants of preventive health actions. To the degree to which the nurse is aware of them, she will be effective in her health promotion role.

A major gap exists between already known methods of prevention and early detection of illness and the public's utilization of these services. For instance, only 40 percent of the women interviewed in a recent nationwide study reported having ever had a Papanicolaou test. Fewer than 10 percent reported having had more than one test(1). Although the number of people using preventive health services has increased from year to year, many others who appear to have adequate knowledge and favorable attitudes about prevention do not always put them into action. Fortunately and appropriately, the expanded role of the professional nurse is now emphasizing those activities that will promote preventive and health maintenance behaviors among the public.

The characteristics of those who use preventive health services have been identified in several studies. They tend to be white, married women who have graduated from college, are in the middle to high income groups, and are members of small families (two to five members)(2). These studies, however, have revealed very little about how to motivate people to take advantage of preventive services.

DR. PENDER, *a graduate of Michigan State University School of Nursing, East Lansing, with her doctorate from Northwestern University, Evanston, Illinois, is an associate professor in the School of Nursing, Northern Illinois University, DeKalb, Illinois.*

Compounding the problem is the fact that many of the persons whom the nurse will be trying to encourage toward more appropriate preventive health behavior will be both physically and psychologically well(3). They must therefore be helped to understand potential rather than actual and immediate health threats. To do this, the nurse herself needs to be aware of the personal, interpersonal, and situational factors that may promote or inhibit preventive health behavior.

PREVENTIVE HEALTH BEHAVIOR DEFINED

A definition of health must serve as the reference point for the nurse concerned with the prevention of illness. One definition is:

> *. . . an asymptomatic state or state of minimal symptoms resulting from biological or cyclical as opposed to pathological changes with evidence of a socially and personally valued functional level in relation to role performance and with a minimum probability of change to a less valued function level*(4).

Kasl and Cobb have identified three types of health-related behaviors. *(Preventive) health behavior* they define as any behavior undertaken for the purpose of preventing disease or detecting disease in an asymptomatic state. *Illness behavior* is any activity undertaken by a person who feels ill, for the purpose of defining the state of his health and discovering a suitable remedy. *Sick-role behavior* is any activity undertaken by a person who considers himself to be sick, for the purpose of getting well again.

Thus, preventive health behavior can be described as individual or group action taken to minimize the potential threat of illness. It is, in most instances, voluntary, its purpose is neither curative nor remedial, and it is performed when an individual is asymptomatic in relation to a specific illness.

Preventive health behavior has two major components—primary prevention and early detection. For some health problems primary prevention measures are available: dietary and weight control, for instance, appropriate exercise and rest patterns, immunization, and the like. For other health problems, however, only early detection techniques—x-ray, Pap smears, thermography, electrocardiograms, glaucoma screening, and the like—can minimize the threat of developing a serious or catastrophic illness.

Preventive health behavior manifests itself in two phases: decision-making and action, with the latter contingent on the former.

DECISION-MAKING PHASE

Personal, interpersonal, and situational factors are the three main determinants in the decision-making phase.

Personal Determinants. Perceptions provide the subjective ideas that serve as the motivating forces toward preventive health behavior. The major personal determinants of such behavior are the individual's perceptions of (1) the importance of health, (2) his own vulnerability, (3) value of early detection, (4) seriousness, (5) efficacy of action, and (6) level of internal versus external control.

Importance of health. In a recent study, Palmore found that life satisfaction in middle age was largely influenced by self-rated health rather than by career anchorage, income, education, or social activity(7). If health is so important to people, then, why isn't there a greater public demand for preventive health services?

The answer may lie in the fact that health does not appear to be valued for its own sake, but rather because it enables people to pursue other objects, relationships, and goals that *are* directly valued. In lessening the threat of illness to himself, the individual ensures his ability to enjoy eating, sleeping, recreation, and socializing. Thus, health maintenance often stems from nonhealth-related motives.

Perceived vulnerability. An individual's own estimate of the probability that he will encounter a specific health problem is another motivating factor(8). In this respect, family health history is important. The greater the incidence of a specific illness within the family and the closer the blood relationship of the affected persons to an individual, the greater the likelihood of his perceiving his vulnerability as high.

Present health status is another determinant. If the individual considers himself weak or fatigued, he may conclude that he is highly susceptible to a specific health problem or to illness in general.

A person may also identify himself as part of a high-risk group, based on the incidence of a specific health problem within the general population. This factor is often related to age. For instance, a 20-year-old man may perceive his vulnerability to myocardial infarction as low, but his projected vulnerability at 50 may be very high. The time between his present age and period of peak perceived vulnerability will undoubtedly affect his attitude toward preventive health services. Unfortunately, effective prevention must often begin well in advance of the peak period, and further research is needed to indicate the relationship between immediacy of health threat and the predisposition to take preventive action.

Perceived value of early detection. There is some evidence that those who value early detection will seek it and those who don't will not. Thus, Kegeles found that almost 50 percent of the women he interviewed who believed in the benefits of early detection techniques had obtained a Pap smear. Only a little over 25 percent of those who did not believe in the benefits of early detection had obtained the test(1).

Another study has indicated that valuing early detection is illness specific, with different priorities given to various preventive health behaviors(9). Involvement in one form of prevention did not necessarily predict a predisposition to engage in another, although valuing early detection for a specific illness did result in a higher level of readiness to take preventive action in regard to that illness.

Perceived seriousness. Four factors contribute to the perceived seriousness of any given health problem: degree of threat, visibility, degree of alteration in family and occupational roles, and communicability to others. The degree of threat can be conceptualized as a continuum from minimal discomfort through severe discomfort to total disability or death. The emotional arousal experienced by an individual at the thought of a given illness contributes to the threat factor. For instance, "cancer" is an emotionally loaded word associated with a high degree of threat.

Conditions which result in visible physical changes are often considered more serious than less visible problems, since most people value physical attractiveness and social acceptability highly.

Still another component of the perceived seriousness factor is the degree to which a specific illness will interfere with an individual's lifestyle or with the performance of occupational and family roles such as provider, parent, and sexual partner. The value assigned to any given role determines the impact that possible disruption of that role will have on a specific individual.

A fourth aspect of perceived seriousness is the communicability of the illness. While an individual may tolerate personal inconvenience and discomfort, he seldom wishes to endanger the health of family members or friends. His concern for the welfare of others rather than for his own health, then, may motivate him to seek preventive services.

Perceived efficacy of action. An individual is not likely to use preventive services unless he perceives them as effective in lowering the threat of illness. Once he decides to act, he will choose the alternative that he sees as having the highest probability of success with the least amount of risk or inconvenience. Since persons in higher educational or socioeconomic levels may be more aware of the whole range of preventive health alternatives available, they are also more likely than persons in lower educational or socioeconomic levels to choose the most effective ones.

Perceived level of internal versus external control. When a person sees himself as powerless, he believes he has little chance to exert control over his environment—that is, he feels his life is externally controlled. Such feelings often characterize people within the lower socioeconomic class, where the incidence of preventive health behavior is very low.

Kirscht has found that those who are internally controlled view themselves as less vulnerable to ill health but also think preventive health actions are more effective than do externally controlled individuals(10). Thus, those who believe they can influence the course of their own health will use preventive services to a greater extent than those who feel powerless.

Interpersonal Determinants. In addition to the influence that interaction with others has on the personal determinants already discussed, four key interpersonal considerations seem to directly influence the decision-making phase: concern of significant others, family patterns of utilization, expectations of friends, and informational input from health professionals.

Concern of significant others. Families often provide the motivation for a particular member to seek health care. Whether the person involved sees encouragement by his family as loving concern or irritating persistence, he may seek to allay their anxiety because he believes that in doing so he is contributing to the stability of the family. This is another good example of how nonhealth-related motives may result in health-related behavior.

Family patterns of utilization. Patterns of health behavior are developed early in childhood, primarily through imitation, and with parents and teachers usually serving as role models. Tyroler, in studying families' participation in an oral polio vaccine program, found similarity of health behavior within families in both upper and lower socioeconomic groups. Similarity between the behavior of mother and child was high, between husband and wife intermediate, and between father and child relatively low(11).

High maternal influence has also been reported by Steele and McBroom, who found that the level of education of the dominant female within the household correlated highly with the degree of preventive health behavior(9). Thus, both studies suggest that the mother is often the major decision-maker and role model in this regard.

Expectations of friends. In studying the incidence of polio vaccinations for children, Gray found that expectations of friends were powerful motivators for parents. Parents apparently sought vaccinations for their children to fulfill expectations of what "good parents should do"(12).

Information from professionals. Interaction with professionals perceived as having knowledge and expertise often increases readiness to engage in preventive health behavior. Two studies have shown that the greater the credibility of the source, the more persuasive the motivational message. In contrast, when the information source was perceived as lacking expertise, persons reacted negatively toward the message and actively avoided the behavior advocated(13, 14). The competence the public attributes to the nurse will therefore affect their responsiveness to her suggestions in this regard.

Situational Determinants. Situational determinants—among them, cultural acceptance of health behaviors, societal group norms or pressure, and information from nonpersonal sources—also appear to have an effect on preventive health behavior.

Cultural acceptance of health behaviors. In any culture certain health-related behaviors are sanctioned and others are not. Some cultures consider it inappropriate to seek medical attention unless one is seriously ill. In others, such as the American, people react negatively toward a person who complains of discomfort when no definite physical findings are found in a medical examination. It is thus likely that many people do not seek preventive or early detection measures because of the social stigma attached to preoccupation with bodily processes. Instead, they may wait until their symptoms are pronounced or incapacitating before they seek medical attention—a time too late for prevention and often too late for early detection. People will fully use preventive health services only as doing so becomes increasingly recognized as an acceptable, responsible pattern of action.

Societal group norms and pressures. If a person conforms with societal norms, pressure from society as a whole may influence him to act to maintain his health. Compliance provides him with a sense of satisfaction which reinforces the action taken. For instance, considerable societal pressure to discontinue smoking has induced many people to try to discontinue the habit.

Information from nonpersonal sources. All individuals are exposed to some forms of mass communication. Health information, for instance, is a part of both commercials and regular programming on radio and television and of ads and articles in periodicals and newspapers. The information presented varies in accuracy and clarity, and individuals also vary in their ability to interpret the information correctly. Kirscht and Haefner found that after exposure to films on tuberculosis, heart disease, and cancer, people generally perceived themselves as more vulnerable to these diseases and had more confidence in the efficacy of preventive health actions(15).

ACTION PHASE

Once an individual has decided to engage in preventive behavior of one kind or another, a cue is needed to put his decision into action. Cues may be internal, such as the perception of aging and general fatigue, or external, such as interpersonal communications, billboards, advertisements, or the availability of health facilities themselves—that is, passing by a mobile x-ray unit or a diabetic screening clinic.

Another trigger, according to Steele and McBroom, is a personal experience with illness within the previous year, which yields a higher likelihood of preventive health behavior even in areas unrelated to the illness episode(9). These findings suggest that nurses in the hospital and outpatient clinics as well as community health agencies should assume initial responsibility for persuading presently or recently hospitalized patients to take measures to maintain their health.

The intensity of the cue needed to motivate people into action depends on the level of their readiness to act. While moderate to intense stimuli may be needed to trigger preventive behavior in people with low readiness, only mild stimuli may be necessary for others. For instance, a person in a high state of readiness may be motivated to act by simply walking past a diabetic screening clinic.

An overly strong cue may prompt such overwhelming anxiety that it inhibits rather than encourages the person to take the recommended action. The goal is to create anticipatory fear, in which the individual anticipates that a health problem will occur unless he takes action to prevent it.

Barriers to action. Various types of conflict may impede a person from acting. *Approach-avoidance conflict* occurs when a person weighs the value of a preventive action against the high cost, inconvenience, unpleasantness, pain, or upsetting quality of the action. For instance, an individual may want to have a physical examination as a preventive measure, but hesitates to do so because he fears what the physician may find. This type of conflict is frequently encountered when the health measures involved are directed at early detection.

When two methods of prevention may be equally effective and the person can't decide which one to adopt, *approach-approach conflict* is in operation. In another instance, the symptoms of a potential health problem may legitimize a dependency role which the individual enjoys, although preventive behavior would minimize the probability of encountering further discomfort. An *avoidance-avoidance conflict* occurs if the potential health problem is considered unpleasant but the anticipated changes in life-style brought about by preventive health behavior are also viewed as highly undesirable.

If the individual is unable to resolve his conflicts, he will need professional assistance. Without it he will continue to vacillate and may even completely remove himself from the situation, deny the existence of a health threat, and consequently increase his own vulnerability to illness.

THE ROLE OF THE NURSE

The nurse concerned with illness prevention needs an understanding of the factors that prompt or inhibit preventive health behavior. Through such an understanding, she can more clearly differentiate her role in facilitating the decision-making and the action phases of preventive health behavior.

In the decision-making phase, one of the community nurse's major responsibilities is to provide clients with information about the characteristics of high-risk groups for specific health problems and thus promote realistic perception as to their own vulnerability. They should know, for instance, that they are high-risk for breast cancer if they are from families with histories of cancer of one kind or another. As a result, clients may be more willing to take appropriate preventive action such as learning breast self-examination techniques and arranging for more sophisticated diagnostic procedures, as indicated. As pointed out earlier, the nurse's effectiveness in this respect will be influenced by whether or not the client views her as a credible source of health information and on the degree to which a trusting nurse-client relationship has been established.

This same approach can be applied to many potential health problems so that, together, the nurse and client can draw up a "risk profile" on which an overall plan of protective care can be based. The latter can be extended to include a description of present family patterns for using preventive services. This may show that some needs for preventive health care are already being adequately met. For those needs that are not, the nurse can help the client select the measure with the highest probability of success and the least amount of risk and inconvenience.

A protective plan of care is as essential for the nurse responsible for health maintenance of individuals and families as a therapeutic plan of care is for the nurse caring for a hospitalized patient. It provides an organized data base to direct protective nursing actions, defined by Bower as nursing measures that promote health and prevent disease(16).

Since the perceived seriousness of a specific health problem is another determinant of readiness to engage in relevant health behavior, the nurse may need to tell the individual about the possible consequences of the illness for which he appears to be at high risk. In discussing an individual's vulnerability to a specific illness and the serious consequences of it, however, the nurse needs to realize she is increasing his level of anxiety. A moderate amount of anxiety may be motivating, but the nurse should carefully note her client's response in order to avoid creating such fear that he takes no preventive action at all.

Providing the client with information about the various measures he can take to decrease his vulnerability should immediately follow a discussion of his risk status. This will give the client the tools he needs to achieve a sense of control over his own health status and allay his anxiety or stress.

A number of preventive actions can be taken by the nurse on her own without referring the client to other professional services. She can, for example, help the client develop an organized approach for controlling and monitoring his weight; structure a realistic, progressive exercise program; or identify ways of lowering the level of stress within his environment or coping more effectively with stressful situations. The nurse can also provide diabetic, hypertensive, or other screening services on an individual or community-wide basis.

She should also stress to her clients the importance of early detection since, if they value early detection, they will be more likely to seek out and use preventive health services. The nurse can conduct health teaching for families or larger community groups. Appropriate visual aids and discussion guides can be useful in this respect.

A major problem in health promotion is that individuals must be motivated to act in the absence of any immediate threat to their health. The nurse may have to rely heavily on nonhealth-related interpersonal determinants to provide the needed motivation. She may capitalize, for instance, on the client's perceived expectations of friends and the desire to conform to social norms by a comment such as: "I saw your friend, Mrs. Brown, yesterday at the immunization clinic. All her children have received their immunizations." Although she may not be doing so primarily to protect her family's health, the client may then seek immunization for her children because of perceived expectations of peers.

Once a client is ready to use preventive health services, the nurse can structure the environment to provide cues for action. If the individual is ready to act, then telling him of the location of a screening clinic may be enough to stimulate action. Appropriately placed signs throughout the community, notices in newspapers, and radio and television spots should be capitalized on to the fullest extent.

Sometimes the nurse can do very little about such factors as distance, inconvenience, and unpleasantness—frequent barriers to preventive services. But, in many instances, she can use her position as consumer advocate to work for the provision of preventive services within the immediate neighborhood. Some preventive health services, such as instruction on breast self-examination, she can even provide in the client's home. She can also make other services more acceptable by keeping the waiting time at preventive facilities to a minimum and providing a supervised play area for young children.

CONCLUSION

Increasing emphasis is being placed on the prevention of illness within our society. The Health Maintenance Organization (HMO) and Resources Development Act of 1972 clearly shows this trend. But, since even those preventive services already available to the public are underutilized, it is essential that nurses explore their role in promoting health maintenance. Nurses' actions to prevent illness must be based on the identified multiple factors that determine whether a person will use preventive services. The model of preventive health behavior presented in this paper is an attempt to move in that direction.

REFERENCES

1. KEGELES, S. S., AND OTHERS. Survey of beliefs about cancer detection and taking Papanicolaou tests. *Public Health Rep.* 80:815-823, Sept. 1965.
2. U.S. HEALTH SERVICES AND MENTAL HEALTH ADMINISTRATION. *The Utilization of Health Services: Indices and Correlates; a Research Bibliography 1972*, by L. A. Adey and Robert Eichhorn. (DHEW Publication No. (HSM) 73-3003) Washington, D.C., The Services, 1973.
3. WU, RUTH *Behavior and Illness.* Englewood Cliffs, N.J., Prentice-Hall, 1973, p. 90.
4. PATRICK, D. L., AND OTHERS. Toward an operational definition of health. *J. Health Soc. Behav.* 14:6-23, Mar. 1973.
5. KASL, S. V., AND COBB, S. Health behavior, illness behavior, and sick role behavior. Part 1. *Arch. Environ. Health* 12:246-266, Feb. 1966.
6. GREEN, L. W. *Status Identity and Preventive Health Behavior.* Berkeley, University of California School of Public Health, 1970, p. 11.
7. PALMORE, E., AND LUIKART, C. Health and social factors related to life

satisfaction. *J. Health Soc. Behav.* 13:68-80, Mar. 1972.
8. ROSENSTOCK, I. M. Why people use health services. *Milbank Mem. Fund Q.* 44:94-127, July 1966.
9. STEELE, J. L., AND McBROOM, W. H. Conceptual and empirical dimensions of health behavior. *J. Health Soc. Behav.* 13:382-392, Dec. 1972.
10. KIRSCHT, J. P. Perceptions of control and health beliefs. *Can. J. Behav. Sci.* 4:225-237, Mar. 1972.
11. TYROLER, H. A., AND OTHERS. Patterns of preventive health behavior in populations. *J. Health Hum. Behav.* 6:128-140, Fall 1965.
12. GRAY, R. M., AND OTHERS. The effects of social class and friends' expectations on oral polio vaccination participation. *Am. J. Public Health* 56: 2028-2032, Dec. 1966.
13. HEWGILL, M. A., AND MILLER, G. R. Source credibility and response to fear-arousing communications. *Speech Monogr.* 32:95-101, June 1965.
14. POWELL, F. A., AND MILLER, G. R. Social approval and disapproval in anxiety-arousing communications. *Speech Monogr.* 34:152-159, June 1967.
15. KIRSCHT, J. P., AND HAEFNER, D. P. Reactions to a series of fear-arousing messages. IN *Proceedings.* 77th Annual Convention, AAP. Washington, D.C., American Psychological Association, 1969, pp. 343-344.
16. BOWER, F. L. *The Process of Planning Nursing Care: A Theoretical Model.* St. Louis, C. V. Mosby Co., 1972, p. 41.

Section II Assessing the Health Needs and Practices of Client Groups

The articles in this section provide some insights into techniques that can be employed in assessing the health status, belief systems, and care needs of groups of clients within community settings. Such assessment can help to guide community health nurses in planning effective interventions to promote and maintain the health of the clients they serve.

From *Nursing Outlook* 23:365-368, June 1975. Copyright © 1975. AJN Co.

Community Assessment:
An Epidemiological Approach

SALLY E. RUYBAL • ELEANOR BAUWENS • MARI-JOSE FASLA

The inclusion of a systematic method of studying a community health problem broadened the scope of senior students' family-centered experience in community nursing.

In this age of accountability and expanding role of the nurse, the community health nurse (CHN) must be prepared to assess problems, needs, and resources in the community if she is to contribute to the wellness of the families in her caseload. In addition, she must be aware of the network of formal and informal systems within the community in which she works. However, she has often had difficulty in finding appropriate resources in the community, because of her lack of skills in developing an operational framework that would enable her to function efficiently in a place as complex as a community. The result has been a constant manipulation of resources, leading to frustration, unsolved problems for families, loss of time, and increased cost to the agency.

As one means of dealing with this problem, we decided to broaden the scope of our course in community health nursing to include an epi-

MS. RUYBAL *(Deaconess Hospital School of Nursing, Cincinnati, Ohio; M.S., University of Colorado School of Nursing, Denver) is assistant professor and chairperson for undergraduate community health nursing at the University of Arizona College of Nursing, Tucson.* DR. BAUWENS, *a graduate of St. Mary's Hospital School of Nursing, Tucson, received her B.S., M.A., and Ph.D. in anthropology from the University of Arizona, Tucson.* MS. FASLA *received her nursing diploma and B.S. degree in France and her M.S. from the University of California, San Francisco. Both she and Dr. Bauwens are assistant professors at the University of Arizona.*

demiologic approach to the study of not only the family, but the community as well.

There are several ways to define a community. A community may be regarded as a place, a collection of people, a social system, or a "community of solution"(1, 2). The latter concept, as defined by the National Commission on Community Health Services, means that "where health services are concerned, the boundaries of each community are established by the boundaries within which a problem can be defined, dealt with, and solved"(3). In this context, a community might be composed of a specific age group, people with a common diagnosis or health-related problem, or those living in a census tract that has a high morbidity rate. It was our goal, as instructors, to have students identify and study problems within such "communities of solution."

COURSE OBJECTIVES

We believed that this type of learning experience would give students a sound basis for community health nursing practice as well as provide them with a systematic approach toward assessing the community, mobilizing existing health resources, cooperating with other professionals, and utilizing existing resources. This knowledge would then assist them in making sound, confident judgments regarding family and community problems.

Our objectives were: (1) to introduce the student to epidemiological methodology and techniques to assess a community; and (2) to illustrate that CHNs can apply epidemiological concepts in family nursing care and community program planning and evaluation.

After the students' orientation to the concept of a community of solution, they were expected to select and define a community in their own terms and then consult with the instructors as to the feasibility of studying it within the limits of a 10-week course. During this time, they were also working with patients and families through assignments at local public and voluntary agencies.

After a problem within the community under study was identified, the students were assisted in examining the scope of the problem. They sought answers to the "who, where, what, and how" aspects of the problem by collecting pertinent information. Further, the students ascertained the extent of the community's adaptation or adjustment, positive or negative, to the problem—that is, students studied how the people were dealing with the problem.

Many times the solutions extended beyond the boundaries of the community being studied. For instance, the problem of available recreational facilities for a particular area extended into several census tracts.

Sometimes, the students were able to analyze the maladaptive ways communities solved their problems. For instance, in one micro-community people didn't use medical services because of lack of transportation.

The instructors also assisted the students in identifying ways that they could gather data and in selecting resources that were available from various agencies in the community at large. At all times, we attempted to present the students with a systematic way of organizing data for community assessment. Consultation with professionals in the community and review of appropriate literature were encouraged.

METHODS FOR COMMUNITY ASSESSMENT

We reviewed with the students various methods for assessing a community. While many of these are concerned with the community at large, we emphasized the distinctions in studying their identified community. Three main methods were suggested.

1. *Observation.* In order to collect data and describe details, students carried out a "community walk" to get a mental picture of the layout—that is, to make note of the location of churches, stores, schools, better houses, poorer houses, parks, and the like. They also were requested to note whether there were such services as paved streets, transportation facilities, telephones, hospitals, and physician's offices. As a result, the students would become aware of the physical structure of the community as well as the services available. Later, students were asked to make a map of the community—that is, to plot out the community buildings, facilities, houses, and so forth.

2. *Interviews.* A second assessment method was interviews. Students initiated conversations as they walked around the community, to become acquainted with the residents. We encouraged them to take advantage of all locations and situations where informal conversations were likely to occur, such as post offices, street corners, and markets. They contacted individuals too—persons with a specific health problem, typical members of the community being studied, leaders, and so forth—and arranged formal interviews. The first meeting was generally for introductions; the second, for beginning their assessment.

With faculty help, each student outlined a set of questions relating to the 'kinds of things she would like to know about the person or community. These were to serve as a guide for the student; the interviews were to develop the questions outlined.

3. *Surveys.* Since people tend to be uncomfortable when an interviewer rattles off a written list of questions, formal, structured surveys

were not recommended for a general community assessment. However, some students did use the survey method to gather such specific facts as the number of preschool children in an area and the number of houses with indoor plumbing.

STUDENT PROJECTS

The actual processes by which the students achieved the objectives of the learning experience included defining their communities, planning how to gather their data, and identifying one or two problems to pursue in depth. The problem(s) became the focal point for study. After gathering data through one or more of the above methods, the students analyzed the results, formulated conclusions, and suggested recommendations. In some instances, students were able to implement their recommendations. The final step was the evaluation.

Throughout the experience, students consulted both with their instructors and peers. The following are some examples of student projects.

In the planning stage, one student learned that during the summer of 1974 Tucson had experienced a high incidence of shigellosis. Upon further study, she chose as her designated community the census tract where most of the cases were identified. She decided to look at various epidemiological factors such as housing conditions, ethnic composition, educational level, employment rates, and income to try to determine the reasons for the high incidence of the disease in this particular area. Observation was used as the main method of assessment. Blocks in the census tract were observed and mapped.

The student found that houses in the area were fairly close together. She also found from census figures for the year 1970 that the number of persons per household was 4.4 in this community as compared with 3.0 for the city of Tucson as a whole. Seventy percent of the residents were Mexican-American. The median number of years of school completed was 8.4 as compared with 12.4 for the city. In addition, slightly over 4 percent of the male labor force were unemployed as compared with 3 percent for the county. The percentage of families with an income below the poverty level was more than double that for the city.

The student concluded that such factors as crowded living conditions, a low education and income level, and a high unemployment rate did play a part in this community's high incidence of shigellosis. When she consulted with officials from the local health department, she found that a study done on the disease in Tucson revealed that many families who contracted shigellosis were Mexican-Americans who had recently visited in Mexico.

The student recommended that educational programs be instituted in the schools in this area regarding the communicability of shigellosis and methods to prevent the spread of the disease. She visited the local public school and shared her information with the school nurse. She also suggested that pamphlets be prepared for parents both in English and Spanish.

Another student, because of her interest, was assigned to one Yaqui Indian family living 12 miles outside the city limits in the new Pascua Village. Some 750 Yaqui families had been relocated in a new housing development in the village from an inner city ghetto. The student's objective was to study—through direct observation, albeit in a limited way—the mores and habits of the Mexican-Indian culture represented by this group of families.

She found that many hardships for that population had been alleviated by the move but new ones were created as well. Health care—a very vital need of this new growing population—was inaccessible because of lack of transportation to medical facilities in the city.

Theoretically, there are two ways to correct the problem: (1) bring the people to existing health care facilities, or (2) bring the facilities to the people.

From a survey of the literature, including newspapers, and from a series of formal and informal interviews with people living in the village and those working for the Yaqui Indians, a descriptive study emerged. The students investigated what had been attempted to date to alleviate the problem, either by providing transportation to the health care facilities or by providing direct health services to the people in their community. She looked at the present strengths and weaknesses inside and outside the community and possible resources to meet the health needs of this population. Among other things, she studied the lack of public transportation to and from this area, looked at the alternatives, and made some recommendations.

A BRIDGE OF COMMUNICATION

The most practical and feasible one was to have a permanent, full-time satellite clinic located within the village with direct linkage to acute care facilities in Tucson. It was further recommended that community members be involved as health workers in this satellite clinic. This would create a bridge of communication and understanding between the clinic and the Yaqui population. The clinic would become an integral part of the village life. She made her recommendations known through her talks with interested people and was informed that they were passed on to a health official involved with rural health in the state.

Two students accepted the challenge of a community assessment project involving the local chapter of the Muscular Dystrophy Association. The students initially assessed the local situation—the epidemiology of muscular dystrophy in a city of approximately 400,000 population. They looked into existing resources and analyzed which were being utilized and which were underutilized. They became involved with schools, local voluntary .agencies, and state and national associations. This led to their attending meeting of local parent muscular dystrophy groups.

After attending several local group meetings, the students soon started identifying a different level of problems. These were very practical everyday problems that parents and families face when a member has a degenerative chronic disease. The students found that parents caring for children with this disease were encountering many mental health problems.

One resource not available to these families was support in coping with the afflicted member. As a solution, the students initiated a program of volunteer "home relief workers" to assist with the physical and emotional care of the patient. This gave the other family members time to engage in activities to meet their own needs. The volunteer relief workers were recruited via the public media with students appearing for TV and radio public service announcements.

To help prepare the volunteers for their responsibilities, students collaborated with physiotherapists at a local medical center. Physical skills that involved using a Hoyer lift and moving and transferring patients were taught by the students. After the workers had been trained, their names were placed on a list at the local muscular dystrophy nursing office and were available to families in need of a qualified helper.

This exercise in community assessment enabled the student to (1) analyze existing resources, (2) develop a system of resources and personnel, and (3) become involved with a local group and solve a problem of its members.

Using this epidemiologic approach, the students were able to put the objectives of the learning experience into operation. As a result of the students' efforts, the local muscular dystrophy chapter donated a film about MD to the college of nursing and made the students honorary members of the chapter.

Other student projects included examining local emergency transportation problems, studying the attitudes of health personnel toward Mexican-American patients in an emergency clinic of a county hospital, exploring the causes of the high incidence of infant mortality in a particular area of the city, relating environmental factors to the incidence of tuberculosis, and studying housing for the elderly.

EVALUATING THE EXPERIENCE

The students presented their final reports, both verbal and written, in class seminar. The criteria used for evaluating their work were:

- clarity of the definition and profile of the community
- description of the environmental factors within the family unit and community, using epidemiological data
- demonstration of the use of professional consultants and evidence of professional literature read
- quality of results of using the tools and methods of assessment
- presentation of findings and specific problems identified
- recommendations regarding the CHN's health responsibility and role
- recommendations for further action.

The presentations demonstrated that the students gained the ability to identify problems in the community. Students were also able to interpret the responsibilities and role of the community health nurse in reducing environmental health hazards (shigella epidemic) and in changing either some aspects of the environment (playgrounds) or some condition of people in the community (muscular dystrophy). Also, the projects reflected to some extent the students' ability to be more observant and perceptive of problems, needs, and resources in the community.

As faculty, we too were interested in the outcomes of the learning experience. Specifically, we wanted to know if the two main objectives of the course were met—had the students learned epidemiological methods and techniques to assess a community and were they able to apply them to a specific situation. The student projects indicated a positive application of epidemiologic methodology to family and community assessment. The students demonstrated that they were able to go into the community and collect data in a more systematic way than previously. This type of learning experience encouraged creativity and independence in the students and broke the routine of having to write a family analysis paper at the completion of the community health nursing course. It offered the student an alternative for synthesizing and crystallizing knowledge.

The experience not only generated innovative ideas for faculty in teaching community health nursing, but it also provided a way of enriching the students' involvement in their own learning. In other words, we brought "Pygmalion" to the classroom. For most students, community nursing suddenly became dynamic and relevant to the delivery of health care. The students' enthusiasm created excitement among themselves, uninvolved students, and other faculty. More specifically, we learned that student involvement in setting up the learning experience is imperative to success. Also, we found a way of bringing what the community has to offer to the academic classroom and discovered that epidemiology can be taught as a framework for family and community nursing practice.

REFERENCES

1. SANDERS, I. T. The community structure and function. *Nurs. Outlook* 11:642-646, Sept. 1963.
2. NATIONAL COMMISSION ON COMMUNITY HEALTH SERVICES. *Health Is a Community Affair.* Cambridge, Mass., Harvard University Press, 1966, pp. 2-4.
3. Ibid.

From *Nursing Research* 25:433-439, Nov.-Dec. 1976. Copyright © 1976. AJN Co.

Health Needs of the Elderly

SISTER MARY JEANNE HAIN • SHU-PI C. CHEN

Elderly residents in two high-rise apartments in Erie, Pennsylvania, were surveyed to identify health needs in this type of congregate dwelling.

Although increasing numbers of elderly persons are moving into high-rise apartments, health needs of these residents have not been documented to any extent. This study attempted to identify health needs of the elderly in two high-rise apartments for senior citizens in Erie, Pennsylvania.

Background of the Study. One of the most prevalent myths about old people is that large numbers of them live in institutions. Actually, only five percent of older people reside in such settings. Ninety-five percent are on their own in the community, living either by themselves or with spouse, family, or friends(1). Through a combination of private and public resources, an increasingly wide range of choice in living arrangements is being offered to the elderly. Income is often the key factor. Low-cost public housing and government-aided housing developed by churches, unions, or other nonprofit groups are available(2). Living independently in apartments can be possible if medical services and ready access to hospital facilities are provided(1).

Eighty-six percent of the elderly have chronic health problems of one

SISTER MARY JEANNE HAIN *(Spencer Hospital School of Nursing, Meadville, Pennsylvania: M.S., University of Illinois, Chicago) is an assistant professor of nursing—adult health instructor, Erie Institute for Nursing, Villa Maria College, Erie, Pennsylvania.* SHU-PI C. CHEN *(University of California, Los Angeles School of Nursing; Dr. P. H., University of California, Los Angeles, School of Public Health) is associate professor in the Department of Public Health Nursing. College of Nursing, University of Illinois at the Medical Center, Chicago.*

kind or another that require more frequent doctor visits, more and longer hospital stays, as well as more periods of illness at home which may result in more physical and emotional disability(1). The most frequently reported activity-limiting conditions are cardiovascular (21.8 percent), arthritic (20.7 percent), and visual problems (9.5 percent)(3). Many old people lack the skills and energy to overcome the barriers to adequate health care. Some elderly persons believe the symptoms of illness are normal and inevitable results of aging and do not seek help. Others are aware of their need for help but lack the knowledge or energy required to reach available services(4).

Indicators. Health needs in this study were defined in relation to three indicators: health condition, physical functioning, and access to medical care. These indicators were used in the DuPage, Illinois County Health Department survey(5). Health condition included number of days of illness, status of ambulation, and difficulty with symptoms during the month prior to interview. Physical functioning indicated capacity during the month prior to interview in five activities of daily living adapted to the apartment setting: getting about in the apartment; doing own laundry; washing, bathing, dressing, putting on shoes (self-care factors); getting around outside apartment complex; and cutting toenails(6). Access to medical care included situations of emergency, non-emergency, and routine health care.

Method. *Setting.* The community of Erie, Pennsylvania, after considering housing problems for senior citizens, built high-rise apartments. At the time of the study, the number of elderly persons over 65 years of age was approximately 14,000, of which two-thirds were women. Four apartment complexes were planned for this age group, but only two were in operation at the time of the study. Criteria for admission to these dwellings were annual incomes of not more than $5,200 and independence on the part of the residents. No provisions were made for medical services. One high-rise apartment, established for those with low incomes, had been in operation for two and one-half years; this residence is located two blocks from the city's main street. The other, located six miles out of the city off Lake Erie and surrounded by beautiful grounds, is designated a residence for moderate-income elderly. The city also established a Senior Citizens Center located one block from the low-income high-rise.

Population and Sample. The population of this study included all persons 65 years of age and over who had lived in the two high-rise apart-

60

Table 1. Sample (N = 128) by Sex, Age, and Living Status

Age	Living Status						Composition of Pairs by Age and Sex					
	Males Living Alone		Females Living Alone		Pairs		Male Older		Female Older		Two Females	
	N	(%)	N	(%)	N	(%)	N	(%)	N	(%)	N	(%)
65–69	4	(20.0)	11	(15.5)	7	(18.9)	5	(13.5)	2	(5.4)	–	–
70–74	3	(15.0)	19	(26.8)	8	(21.6)	5	(13.5)	3	(8.1)	–	–
75–79	6	(30.0)	24	(33.8)	14	(37.8)	10	(27.0)	3	(8.1)	1	(2.7)
80–84	4	(20.0)	5	(7.0)	4	(10.8)	2	(5.4)	1	(2.7)	1	(2.7)
85+	3	(15.0)	5	(7.0)	4	(10.8)	3	(8.1)	1	(2.7)	–	–
Total	20	(100.0)	71	(100.0)	37	(99.9)	25	(67.5)	10	(27.0)	2	(5.4)
$\bar{X} \pm$ SD	76.3 ± 7.0		75.8 ± 5.4		76.2 ± 5.14		76.4 ± 6.5		74.9 ± 6.8		80.5 ± 2.12	
Range	65–88		66–89		65–91		66–91		65–87		79–82	

ment buildings for at least six months. During July-August 1973, there were 133 households in the moderate-income high rise and 200 households in the low-income apartment building. Of the total 333 households, 285 were eligible for inclusion in the study. According to sex and living status, the population consisted of 23 men living alone, 224 females living alone, and 38 pairs. (Pairs consisted of married couples or two of the same sex living in one apartment.)

The sample design selected all males living alone, all pairs, and one-third of females living alone (randomly selected). The purpose of this design was to increase representation of males in the study population.

Two assumptions were made in the sampling process: 1) the elder member of pairs would be males and 2) health needs of older adults living alone or in pairs might differ.

The resultant procedure yielded a sample size of 137, including 23 males living alone, 38 pairs, and 76 females living alone. A sampling loss of nine occurred—three elderly not contacted and six refusals, giving a response rate of 94 percent. Thus, the sample size was reduced to 128; 20 males living alone, 37 pairs, and 71 females living alone. Table 1 gives the age, sex, and living status of the sample.

Instrument. A 20-item questionnaire was developed for this study, following the basic structure and rationale of the questionnaire developed for the DuPage study(5). Sample questions for each of the three indicators were:

ACCESS TO MEDICAL CARE:
   If ill during the last month, did you see a doctor?
   Regardless if you are sick or not, do you go to a doctor on a regular basis?
   In the event of a sudden illness, what do you do?

HEALTH CONDITION:
   During the last month, for the most part, were you up and around at home, in a chair, at home in bed, completely bedridden at home, visiting at home of

friend or relative, or in a hospital or nursing home?

During the last month, did you have any difficulty with the following symptoms? (If yes, did you seek medical attention?)

trouble breathing

pains in chest

swelling of ankles or feet

pains in joints or muscles

frequency of urination

dizzy spells

sores that do not heal

trouble hearing

trouble seeing

other

During the last month, how many days were you sick to the point of having to give up some of your regular activities such as visiting, going shopping, or cooking for yourself?

PHYSICAL FUNCTIONING:

I am going to read a list of activities that many people have difficulty with as they grow older. After I read each one, please tell me if you have no difficulty, some difficulty, or whether you cannot do it at all.

1. getting about in the apartment
2. doing own laundry
3. washing, bathing, dressing, putting on shoes
4. getting around outside apartment complex
5. cutting your own toenails

In addition, nine questions that related to distance traveled for health care, method of transportation used to obtain health care, and cost of health care were asked. A tenth question on the instrument was open-ended, asking the client if there was anything he felt was a problem or a need in his way of life today. Data from these ten questions were not included in the study.

Prior to the 1972 DuPage study, a pretest was conducted to determine congruency in the reporting of health problems by the public health nurses and the older adults who received care. An 87 percent agreement gave the DuPage investigators some assurance that older adults responded to questions consistently with the public health nurses' perception of their health problems. Because of the experience of this study, the content of the Erie study questionnaire was not exclusively tested. However, clarity of the wording of the questionnaire was sought. Two Chicago residents over 65 years of age were interviewed. The respondents indicated they had no difficulty in responding to the questionnaire. The questionnaire was also sent to three Erie residents who were over 65 years of age, but resided in their own homes. These respondents also indicated they had no difficulty in responding to the questionnaire. Based on these five trial cases, the questionnaire was finalized and a coding system was developed. Reliability and validity, though not statistically established, were assumed.

Data Collection. Rules observed during data collection were: One of the two authors was designated to collect all data. Although this did not eliminate interviewer bias, it could be assumed the bias was unidirectional. If an elderly person was unable to be reached or refused to participate, no substitute was chosen. If an elderly person was unable to respond to the interview, a relative of the person was asked to be a proxy respondent. When two elderly persons lived in one household, the older was selected as the study subject. When the respondent was not at home at the time of the initial contact, at least four additional attempts were made to reach him.

The interviewer introduced herself to the person who answered the door, according to an established formula. After locating the head of the household, the interviewer read the 20 items from the prepared questionnaire to the respondent and wrote in the answers. The respondent was asked to limit answers to activities and experiences of the last month(7).

Data Analysis. A dichotomy technique yielding an indicator for health condition, physical functioning, and access to medical care was used to identify the health needs. Professional judgment, based on the authors' knowledge and experiences in clinical nursing, was used to classify the dichotomy.

For health condition, according to the dichotomy of well and not well. if the illness lasted one to seven days, the condition was considered minor; respondents who reported up to seven days of illness were judged to be well persons. Ambulatory status was reflected by respondents' ability to walk, ranging from up and round, visiting, or being home in bed. Elderly who reported ability to visit or be up and around at home and outside were judged well persons; elderly who responded to any other degree of ambulation such as up and around at home only or help with ambulation were judged not well. Nine symptoms known to cause problems among older adults, selected through literature review(5) and professional experience, were: trouble hearing, pains in joints or muscles, pains in chest, trouble seeing, trouble breathing, frequency of urination, dizzy spells, swelling of feet or ankles, and sores that do not heal. If a respondent reported having difficulty with five or more symptoms listed above, he was judged to be not well. The health condition indicator was developed by judging well and not well responses to the three questions.

To measure physical functioning, the elderly were asked to indicate degree of difficulty in the five activities of daily living; no difficulty, some difficulty, or cannot do it. Using a well-not well dichotomy, elderly who responded to no difficulty in one activity were considered well. If elderly indicated one of the other two responses, they were not well.

Access to medical care was studied from interview responses regarding visits to a physician if the respondent had been ill during the month prior to interview (referred to as nonemergency situation), respondents' seeking routine health care, and respondents' actions in event of an emergency. Three interpretations by the authors were given to the interview responses for each of the three medical care situations: respondent had access (Y), respondent did not have access (N), authors were uncertain from the responses given to the situation (U).

Data were coded and transferred for data processing. Verification of data was carried out by using computer program BMDO4D(8).

The chi-square test was used, and level of significance was set at .05. In examining the results, two facts should be kept in mind: sampling loss was 13 percent (323) for males living alone, 6.6 percent (576) for females living alone, and 2.6 percent (138) for pairs. Pairs consisted of 25 male and 12 female respondents.

Results. A difference in response between residents of the two high-rises was noted. Low-income residents were suspicious, questioned the interviewer as to whether she was working for the state or one of the local hospitals, frequently asking where the information was going and whether it really was confidential. In the moderate-income high-rise, many residents identified the interviewer with their children or grandchildren who had conducted similar exercises in their educational process.

Health Condition. Health condition was studied from interview responses regarding number of days elderly were ill to the point of having to give up regular activities, ambulation status, and difficulty with symptoms one month prior to interview.

Table 2 lists the frequency and percentage distribution of the eight patterns of health condition indicators observed in the three sub-samples. Further, to derive one indicator for health condition, professional judgment was applied. For example, an elderly person who reported less

Table 2. Frequency and Percentage Distributors of Health Condition Indicator of Three Subsamples

Pattern No.	Health Condition				Subsample							
	Indicator	General Health	Ambulation	Symptoms	Males Living Alone		Females Living Alone		Pairs		Total	
					N	(%)	N	(%)	N	(%)	N	(%)
1.	W¹	W	W	W	17	(85.0)	41	(57.7)	23	(62.2)	81	(63.3)
2.	W	W	W	NW	–	–	8	(11.3)	2	(5.4)	10	(7.8)
3.	W	W	NW	W	–	–	2	(2.8)	3	(8.1)	5	(3.9)
4.	W	NW	W	W	–	–	1	(1.4)	–	–	1	(0.8)
				Subtotal	17	(85.0)	52	(73.2)	28	(75.7)	97	(75.8)
5.	NW¹	W	NW	NW	–	–	4	(5.6)	–	–	4	(3.1)
6.	NW	NW	W	NW	–	–	2	(2.8)	–	–	2	(1.6)
7.	NW	NW	NW	W	3	(15.0)	11	(15.5)	6	(16.21)	20	(15.6)
8.	NW	NW	NW	NW	–	–	2	(2.8)	3	(8.1)	5	(3.9)
				Subtotal	3	(15.0)	19	(26.7)	9	(24.3)	31	(24.3)
				Total	20	(100.0)	71	(99.9)	37	(100.0)	128	(100.0)

¹W = well: NW = not well

than seven days of illness (W), did not report being confined to bed or hospitalized, was able to ambulate without help (W), and reported difficulty with less than five symptoms (W) was assigned a health condition of well. On the contrary, an elderly person who reported more than eight days of illness (NW), confinement to bed (NW), help needed with ambulation (NW), or hospitalization and difficulty with five or more symptoms (NW) was assigned a not well health condition. Thus, among the eight patterns, health condition patterns 1, 2, 3, 4 were well; the remaining were not well (Table 2). The chi-square test of homogeneity yielded no significant differences among the three subsamples regarding health condition (x^2 = 1.176, df = 2, $p < .60$). However, data revealed 24.3 percent of the elderly surveyed were not well (Table 2). Males living alone had more difficulty with pains in chest. Females living alone had more difficulty with swelling of feet and ankles and dizzy spells. Pains in joints or muscles ranked first or second in all three subsamples. Of the three subsamples, pairs had the highest percentage of hospitalization and confinement.

Table 3. Frequency and Percentage Distributions of Physical Functioning Indicator of Three Subsamples

Pattern No.	Indicator	Activities					Subsample							
		Getting About Apt.	Doing Laundry	Self Care	Getting Outside Apt.	Cutting Toenails	Males Living Alone		Females Living Alone		Pairs		Total	
							N	(%)	N	(%)	N	(%)	N	(%)
1.	W¹	W	W	W	W	W	13	(65.0)	30	(42.3)	24	(64.9)	67	(52.3)
2.	W	W	W	W	W	NW	–	–	9	(12.7)	4	(10.8)	13	(10.2)
3.	W	W	NW	W	W	W	1	(5.0)	1	(1.4)	–	–	2	(1.6)
4.	W	W	NW	N	W	NW	3	(15.0)	1	(1.4)	1	(2.7)	5	(3.9)
						Subtotal	17	(85.0)	41	(57.8)	29	(78.4)	87	(68.0)
5.	NW¹	NW	W/NW	W/NW	W/NW	W/NW	3	(15.0)	12	(16.9)	6	(16.2)	21	(16.4)
6.	NW	W/NW¹	W/NW	NW	W/NW	W/NW	–	–	4	(5.6)	1	(2.7)	5	(3.9)
7.	NW	W/NW	W/NW	W/NW	NW	W/NW	–	–	14	(19.7)	1	(2.7)	15	(11.7)
						Subtotal	3	(15.0)	30	(42.2)	8	(21.6)	41	(32.0)
						Total	20	(100.0)	71	(100.0)	37	(100.0)	128	(100.0)

¹W = well. NW = not well. W/NW = well or not well

Physical Functioning. The physical functioning indicator was determined by the authors, based on their professional judgment regarding the levels of ability in physical functioning activities. If a response was not well in getting about in the apartment, the indicator was classified as not well regardless of responses in the other four activities, i.e., pattern five. If a response was not well in self-care, the indicator was not well, regardless of the other responses, i.e., pattern six. If a response was not well in getting around outside apartment, the indicator was not well regardless of the other responses, i.e., pattern seven (Table 3). A chi-square test of homogeniety yielded a result among the three subsamples ($x^2 = 7.913$, df = 2, $p < .025$). Females living alone had more difficulty with physical functioning, especially in getting about in the apartment, self-care, and getting around outside the apartment. Males living alone had significantly less difficulty with physical functioning.

Access to Medical Care. To develop an indicator for access to medical care, the rules of priorities were: If respondent had access to non-emergency care and routine health care, he was considered to have access to medical care, i.e., patterns one and two. If a respondent had no access to nonemergency care and routine health care, he was considered to have no access to medical care. If a respondent's access to non-emergency and routine health care was questionable (U), i.e., pattern five, his access to medical care was questionable. Emergency care was not given serious consideration in developing the indicator, because the client would not rely on this type of care for maintenance or preventive care. The chi-square test of homogeneity indicated that the proportion of access to medical care did not differ among the three subsamples ($x^2 = 4.522$, df = 2, $p < .20$). All males living alone had access to medical

Table 4. Frequency and Percentage Distribution of Access to Medical Care Indicator by Three Subsamples

Pattern No.	Indicator	Medical Care Situations			Subsample							
		Non-Emergency	Routine Health Care	Emergency	Males Living Alone		Females Living Along		Pairs		Total	
					N	(%)	N	(%)	N	(%)	N	(%)
1.	Y¹	Y	Y/N/U¹	Y/N/U	2	(10.0)	13	(18.3)	5	(13.5)	20	(15.6)
2.	Y	N/U¹	Y	Y/N/U	18	(90.0)	50	(70.4)	25	(67.6)	93	(72.7)
			Subtotal		20	(100.0)	63	(88.7)	30	(81.1)	113	(88.3)
3.	N¹	N		Y/N/U	–	–	1	(1.4)	–	–	1	(0.8)
4.	N	U	N	Y/N/U	–	–	2	(2.8)	1	(2.7)	3	(2.3)
			Subtotal		–	–	3	(4.2)	1	(2.7)	4	(3.1)
5.	U¹	U	U	Y/N/U	–	–	5	(7.0)	6	(16.2)	11	(8.6)
			Total		20	(100.0)	71	(99.9)	37	(100.0)	128	(100.0)

¹Y = yes. N = no. U = uncertain. N/U = no or uncertain. Y/N/U = yes, no, or uncertain

care in contrast to 88.7 percent of females living alone and 81.1 percent of pairs (Table 4). Regarding responses to nonemergency situations, of the 20 males living alone, one was ill and saw a doctor, two were ill but did not consult a doctor, and 17 were not ill. Of the 71 females living alone, 13 were ill and saw a doctor, 9 were ill but did not see a doctor, and 49 were not ill. Of the 37 pairs, 5 were ill and saw a doctor, 7 were ill and did not see a doctor, and 25 were not ill. Thus, of the total group, 19 (17 percent) were ill and saw a doctor, 18 (13 percent) were ill but did not see a doctor, and 91 (70 percent) were not ill. A number of reasons were given why subjects sought routine health care. For all three subsamples, the most prevalent reason for seeking medical care was hypertension, heart condition, arthritis, diabetes, yearly physical, and genitourinary conditions. The reasons for not seeking routine health care were: Subjects did not feel the need, were not satisfied with medical resources, and were physically unable to get to medical care resources.

Subjects' responses regarding emergency situations indicated they were well informed and prepared for emergencies. However, differences between females and males studied regarding action taken in emergency situations were noteworthy: Males living alone called for an ambulance first, while females living alone called relatives or friends.

Patterns of the Three Indicators. Indicators of health condition, physical functioning, and access to medical care were combined to derive eight patterns describing health needs of elderly residing in two high-rise apartments in Erie, Pennsylvania (Table 5). Pattern one indicated 80 percent of males living alone, 47.9 percent of females living alone, and 56.8 percent of pairs were well in health condition, physical functioning, and had access to medical care. On the contrary, pattern eight indicated 1.4 percent of females living alone and 2.7 percent of pairs were not well in health condition or physical functioning and had no access to medical care.

Table 5. Patterns of Health Condition, Physical Functioning, and Access to Medical Care by Three Subsamples

Pattern No.	Indicators			Subsamples							
	Health Condition	Physical Functioning	Access to Medical Care	Males Living Alone		Females Living Alone		Pairs		Total	
				N	(%)	N	(%)	N	(%)	N	(%)
1.	W[1]	W	Y[1]	16	(80.0)	34	(47.9)	21	(56.8)	71	(55.5)
2.	W	W	N[1]	–	–	5	(7.0)	6	(16.2)	11	(8.6)
3.	W	NW[1]	Y	1	(5.0)	13	(18.3)	1	(2.7)	15	(11.7)
4.	W	NW	N	–	–	1	(1.4)	–	–	1	(0.8)
5.	NW	W	Y	1	(5.0)	2	(2.8)	2	(5.4)	5	(3.9)
6.	NW	W	N	–	–	–	–	–	–	–	–
7.	NW	NW	Y	2	(10.0)	15	(21.1)	6	(16.2)	23	(18.0)
8.	NW	NW	N	–	–	1	(1.4)	1	(2.7)	2	(1.6)
			Total	20	(100.0)	71	(99.9)	37	(100.0)	128	(100.1)

[1]W = well, NW = not well, Y = yes, N = no

Discussion. Recommendations for meeting health needs identified by the patterns follow: Pattern one (Table 5) indicates the need to maintain or improve the good health of 55.5 percent of the elderly surveyed. This could be done through health education and screening programs offered at the Senior Citizens' Building. Pattern five indicates 3.9 percent of the elderly were not well in health condition, were well in physical functioning, and had access to medical care. It indicates the need for health monitoring programs to maintain the subjects' general health. For patterns one and five, a nurse practitioner supervising health education, screening, and monitoring programs would be feasible.

Pattern seven indicates 18.0 percent of the elderly surveyed were not well in health condition and physical functioning, but had access to medical care. The most helpful means would be to bring health services to them. A nurse practitioner could assess them in their apartments and make the necessary referrals. Patterns three, four, seven, and eight indicate that 32.1 percent of the elderly surveyed needed assistance in physical functioning. Particularly, ambulatory activities presented more difficulty to females living alone, who also voiced problems in regard to walking outside the apartment complex, managing curbs, getting on and off buses. This could be attributed to physical impairments from arthritis, dizzy spells, or poor eyesight. A home health aide could provide this assistance, or community groups. Cutting toenails caused most difficulty. This finding was consistent with Shanas *et al*(6). A chiropodist visits both high-rise apartments studied which is an advantage that could not be easily provided in private homes.

Patterns two, four, and eight indicate 11.0 percent of elderly surveyed had no access to medical care. Again, a nurse practitioner could assess their health status and make appropriate referrals. Regarding reasons for not seeking care, the most frequent reason was the respondents did not feel the need(9). Thus, the range of health services required by elderly living in high-rise apartments can be effectively organized by identifying their health needs. Some require one type of service while others require more than one as demonstrated in the pattern of indicators.

Health Conditions. Conditions which consistently caused elderly to seek routine health care were hypertension, heart conditions, diabetes, and arthritis. These data can be used to plan the screening, monitoring, rehabilitation, and educational programs needed at the Senior Citizens' Center. Since inability to hear caused so much difficulty in two of the subsamples, types of hearing loss could be evaluated and decisions made whether intervention would be helpful. Many respondents thought the hearing loss was a normal part of the aging process and did nothing about the loss. Prevalence of hearing impairment, arthritis, hypertension, and heart conditions was similar to that reported in a survey of non-institutionalized elderly from the National Center of Health Statistics(4). Therefore, it can be concluded the health conditions which affected the elderly surveyed were no different from those which afflicted other noninstitutionalized elderly.

Physical Functioning. The DuPage County study reported 89 percent of older adults had minimal or no difficulty, whereas in this study 68 percent of the elderly surveyed had minimal or no difficulty (Table 3). The difference could result from different scoring methods or from the fact that the nature of high-rise dwellings attract elderly having limitations in physical functioning. The percentage reports of difficulty among the three subsamples showed a statistical difference (Table 3). Shanas *et al.* also found that single or widowed women were most seriously incapacitated(6). Although older women reside in high-rise apartments, the difficulties in carrying out activities of daily living are the same as other noninstitutionalized elderly women. One advantage to living in high-rise apartments is that older women do not have to walk up and down stairs. Physical functioning was found to be different between male and female respondents in two aspects: doing laundry and getting around outside the apartment. Doing laundry is a female-oriented task. Females living alone and in pairs reported this activity caused the least amount of difficulty, while males living alone reported it caused most difficulty. On the other hand, males traditionally went outside the home as the wage earners while females stayed at home; it was not surprising to learn that females living alone indicated they had more difficulty getting around outside the apartment complex while males living alone enjoyed this activity. Many male respondents made it a point to walk as a form of daily exercise. Shanas *et al.* reported a marked difference in mobility of older men and women. Older women are more likely to be housebound than older men; they are also more likely to report difficulties in getting about(6). The results of this research project found no contradiction to this established theory. Cutting toenails had been reported as first or second in activities causing most difficulty for elderly. This finding was consistent with Shanas *et al.* who reported that difficulty in care of feet are two or three times as common among old people as other self-care factors(6). This may be attributed to reported difficulties with arthritis, poor eyesight, or development of hard nails with the aging process.

Subjects frequently voiced preference for those services close to the residence, especially for those within walking distance. This coincided with a study done by Niebanck, who found that facilities used by elderly residing in senior citizen housing developments should be within certain walking distance of the residence. For each of the several facilities, he recorded a "critical distance" between the residence and facility, beyond which dissatisfactions were expressed by housing occupants(10).

Access to Medical Care. Only 11.7 percent of the elderly surveyed did not have access to medical care or the access to medical care was uncertain (see Table 4). Of the three indicators, the smallest percent of problems were reported in access to medical care(5). The elderly studied for the most part were healthy. Since the high-rises studied provide no medical services and independence on the part of the elderly is an admission criterion, these findings were consistent with a report from the White House Conference on Aging that people who move into an apartment complex with medical services provided tend to be less healthy than those who move into one without such services(11).

Further study of the influence of the high-rise apartment environment on psychologic, social, and personal changes in the elderly are needed. Barrett suggested today's tendency to ghettoize the old destroys the human ecologic balance where people of all ages live in harmony, mutually supportive of all things(12).

Regarding Methodology. The use of dichotomy technique was helpful in identifying health needs. Three difficulties were encountered in conducting the survey: overcoming the suspicions of the respondents, finding sample individuals since they were involved in a variety of activities, and hearing impairments on the part of the respondents.

As study of data progressed, it was interesting to note the difference between males and females living alone, although little inference could be made regarding females and males not living alone because of the masking effect of pairs. Therefore, it is recommended that future studies use the following four cells: females living alone, males living alone, males not living alone, and females not living alone.

Limitations of the Study. There was a 94 percent response rate with a sampling loss of only nine elderly. The sampling loss included three not contacted and six refusals. The not contacted included two males living alone who were hospitalized and one female living alone who was staying with a daughter because of a fractured ankle. The refusals included one pair, one male living alone, and four females living alone. After observation and discussion with the refusals and their neighbors, the interviewer concluded the refusals appeared to be healthy. The interviewer felt that suspicions about the purpose of the study influenced the responses of the refusals. However, the effect of the sampling loss of the two males living alone who were sick and hospitalized during the data collection process may have influenced the results of the subsample of males living alone.

REFERENCES

1. BUTLER, R. AND LEWIS, M. I. *Aging and Mental Health; Positive Psychosocial Approaches,* St. Louis, C. V. Mosby Co., 1973.
2. U.S. PUBLIC HEALTH SERVICE. *Working with Older People. Volume I. The Practitioner and the Elderly.* (Publication No. 1459. Vol. 1, rev. Mar. 1969) Washington, D.C., U.S. Government Printing Office, 1969.
3. _____. *Working with Older People. Volume II. The Biological, Psychological and Sociological Aspects of Aging.* (Publication No. 1459 Vol. 2. Apr. 1970) Washington, D.C., U.S. Government Printing Office, 1970.
4. _____. *Working with Older People. Volume III. The Aging Person: Needs and Services.* (Publication No. 1459 Vol. 3, July 1970) Washington, D.C., U.S. Government Printing Office, 1970.
5. MANAGAN, DOROTHY, AND OTHERS. Older adults: A community survey of health needs. *Nurs Res* 23:426-432, Sept.-Oct. 1974.
6. SHANAS, ETHEL AND OTHERS. *Old People in Three Industrial Societies.* New York, Atherton Press, 1968.
7. U.S. NATIONAL CENTER FOR HEALTH STATISTICS. VITAL AND HEALTH STATISTICS. *Health Survey Procedure.* (Series 1 no. 2) Washington, D.C., U.S. Government Printing Office, 1964.
8. DIXON, W. J., ED. *BMD Biomedical Computer Programs.* Los Angeles, University of California Press, 1973.
9. SHANAS, ETHEL. *The Health of Older People.* Cambridge, Mass., Harvard University Press, 1962.
10. NIEBANCK, P. L. *The Elderly in Older Urban Areas.* Philadelphia, Institute for Environmental Studies, University of Pennsylvania, 1965.
11. WHITE HOUSE CONFERENCE ON AGING, 1971. *Toward a National Policy on Aging-Volume I.* Washington, D.C., U.S. Government Printing Office, 1973.
12. BARRETT, J. H. *Gerontological Psychology.* Springfield, Ill., Charles C. Thomas Publisher, 1972.

From *MCN The American Journal of Maternal Child Nursing* 21:168-173, May-June 1977.

Mexican-American Folk Beliefs: How They Affect Health Care

IRENE F. ABRIL

Repudiating traditional cultural ideas about health will succeed only in alienating patients and re-affirming any resentments they have against the Anglo health care system. Rather, we must blend new with old in care that is effective and acceptable to patients.

Anthropological studies indicate the importance of understanding cultures aside from the dominant one if health professionals are to attain a positive outcome in dealing with people from various backgrounds. The Spanish-speaking migrant population of the Southwest is one group of people whose folk beliefs and customs affect their acceptance of health supervision, care, and maintenance.

In considering the culture of the Spanish-speaking population in this area of the country it is important to identify three major subgroups: Spanish-Americans, who are descendants of families living in the Southwest for several hundred years; Mexican-Americans, who are native-born descendants of families who migrated from Mexico (largely since 1910); and citizens of Mexico or recent immigrants(1).

Each of these subgroups has its own cultural ways, beliefs, and historical background. Due to interaction and intermarriage, however, they all have cultural similarities. Thus, in this article "Mexican-American" will encompass all three groups.

The degree to which folk beliefs and practices are accepted varies with Mexican-Americans—particularly from generation to generation—and is largely dependent on education and extent of acculturation. Many attitudes and practices have, however, filtered down through the years, becoming diluted, and are now considered "traditional" to even fourth or fifth generation individuals. Among these are their attitudes toward health and illness.

PERCEPTIONS OF HEALTH AFFECTING CARE

Mexican-Americans perceive illness as a state of physical discomfort. Their most common criteria of good health are a sturdy body, the ability to maintain a high level of normal physical activity, and the absence of persistent pain and discomfort. Therefore, if a person has no outward symptoms as in early anemia, tuberculosis, or heart disease, he is believed to be well and healthy. Similarly, prevention is a concept with which Mexican-Americans have difficulty. This situation may prove to be a challenge to the nurse who is counseling a patient on the importance of early treatment and prevention.

Furthermore, Mexican-Americans often have poor understanding of ideas about germs and contagious disease. They have their own beliefs about the causes of disease. One common belief is that many illnesses occur because of God's displeasure with an individual's behavior. *Seya por Dios* (It is God's will.) is a typical reflection of the Mexican-American regarding any disease state, such as congenital anomaly, which he does not understand.

Accordingly, *mandas* (pledges) to God or a patron saint are made to ensure the welfare of an individual in any dangerous circumstance. This is an especially common practice among pregnant women. The woman may promise, for example, not to cut her infant's hair until a specified age and only after a visit is made to a special chapel or church.

THE FORCES OF NATURE AND THE SUPERNATURAL

Exposure to the forces of nature—such as moonlight, eclipses, cold, heat, air, wind, sun, and water—also are believed to cause illnesses. An example of this is seen in the folk belief of *mal aigre*, which is a cold or "bad" air which affects children and adults, causing pain, cramps, and most commonly facial twitching and paralysis(2). Fearing this ailment, many mothers are hesitant to take their children from a very warm room directly into the cold, especially infants who have just awakened. Keep-

MS. ABRIL, R.N., *is a pediatric nurse associate with the Yuma County Health Department in Arizona. A Mexican-American herself, she works primarily in a well-child clinic, where the majority of clients are from Spanish-speaking migrant worker families. This article was adapted from a version which appeared in Arizona Nurse, the official publication of the Arizona Nurses' Association, May-June 1975. Volume 28, Number 3.*

ing an infant or child partially covered during a physical examination may allay some of the mother's fears about *mal aigre.*

Another example of the influence on health attributed to the forces of nature is the belief that if a pregnant woman is exposed to a lunar eclipse, her infant will be born with a cleft lip and/or palate or with other anomalies. To prevent this from happening, after exposure the woman wears a *cinta* or belt to which a set of keys is attached in such a way that the keys lay right over the womb. She wears the *cinta* until the child's birth. Understanding of this folk belief, explanation of fetal formation *in utero,* alleviation of guilt feelings, and much-needed emotional support are indicated for these mothers.

Brujeria, witchcraft, is regarded as another cause of disease by many Mexican-American people. They believe certain people can cause illness through magical powers. While I was making a home visit as a public health nurse, the maternal grandmother of a 3-year-old with anemia told me that her daughter had died giving birth to the child.

Approximately one month prior to the baby's birth, she said, three *lechusas,* a type of gray owl, had hovered around their small home, made "laughing" sounds, and perched on their porch. The grandmother stated that this was a very bad sign, denoting *mal puesto* or witch's hex. Although her daughter's cause of death was listed as "foreign object in peritoneal cavity," the old woman insisted *brujeria* was responsible. Reporting that her brother had also died of *mal puesto,* she confided that she now lives in fear that perhaps her granddaughter is also hexed.

My nutrition counseling and discussion of anemia failed to allay this woman's fear. I therefore tried to locate and refer to her a *curandera* (healer). The *curandera* is believed to have the power to remove hexes through the use of herbs and prayers.

Mal ojo or evil eye is also a source of illness having magical implications. Small children and infants are thought to be particularly susceptible to its influence. It is believed that if someone, especially a woman, with "strong vision" admires someone else's child, looking at the child without actually touching him, the child may fall ill of *ojo*(2).

The evil power is transmitted through the covetous gaze of that person. Symptoms of the resulting malady include insomnia, aches and pains, excessive crying, fever, severe headache, and restlessness.

The simplest treatment for *ojo* is to have the person who exerted the influence touch the child to break any possible evil bond. Some parents may even expect that person to make the sign of the cross over the child. Many times, however, the person responsible may not be known, as a stranger may have deeply admired the child or infant in a public place. In this case, the treatment procedure becomes much more complex.

If *mal ojo* is suspected, diagnosis is made by rubbing a whole raw egg over the child's body; the egg is then broken open and the yolk examined. A red spot (eye) on the yolk is a diagnostic sign(2). The same egg is put into a small bowl of water and a cross made of blessed palms is laid over it. The bowl is then placed under the head of the victim's bed. This is thought to help draw out the evil force. The following morning the egg is buried, away from plants to avoid the force of any evil from it from wilting them(2).

In intervening when a child has the symptoms of *ojo,* the nurse needs to explain that they can also indicate other illnesses for which there is medicine. The mother should be encouraged to seek medical attention for her child if her own efforts to cure *mal ojo* are unsuccessful.

HOT AND COLD IMBALANCES

Another Mexican-American folk category for illnesses follows the theory of hot/cold imbalance, which originated from the medieval Hippocratic Theory of Pathology. This theory states that illness is due to an imbalance of four body "humours," phlegm, blood, black bile, and yellow bile(2). Likewise, whenever there is an imbalance of hot and cold areas in the body, illness results. Some diseases are "hot" diseases and some "cold." Foods and herbs are also classified into hot and cold for treatments.

If one's feet get wet, for example, it is believed that it is important to get one's head (the fontanel area) wet as well or the imbalance will lead to a sore throat. During the prenatal period a woman may also watch her intake of "hot" foods so as not to affect the fetus adversely. After delivery she may be careful in eating "cold" foods because of the delicate condition of the womb and fear of becoming sterile with a "cold womb." Chili, a hot food, is given to an adult with a cold disease such as pneumonia or a common cold. Similarly, lard, having "cold" properties, is used on burns. Introducing ice for the treatment of burns is usually well accepted by Mexican-Americans because it conforms to these folk beliefs.

Colic is believed caused by a "cold" stomach and is treated by vigorously rubbing the abdomen, and sometimes the back and legs, with olive oil. After this is done, one-half teaspoon of olive oil with a pinch of salt in it is given to the infant. Successful results of this home treatment are high, probably because of its soothing effect on the baby.

Rubbing the soles of the feet with Vicks Vapo-Rub® and giving the child warm herbal teas are thought to balance out the cold disease process of tonsillitis or sore throat. While this home remedy may be soothing and helpful, nursing intervention should include securing a throat culture to rule out the possibility of a strep infection.

Herbs are commonly used for treating "cold" diseases in children and infants as well as for other types of illnesses. *Catarro*, stuffy nose, and *resfriado*, head cold, are both attributed to cold wind and drafts and are treated with herbal teas. Increasing the child's intake of fluids, which we promote for the common cold, can therefore be done within the framework of the Mexican-American culture by encouraging the traditional use of herbal tea.

Among the more common herbs and the conditions for which they are used are those given below. They may be used alone or in combination:

- *Aniz Verde* (anise seed)—used for treating diminishing milk in breast-feeding mothers and for patients suffering with asthma and bronchitis.
- *Rose de Castillo* (rose petals)—used for prevention of swelling of the eyes; for reducing fever; and as a diuretic.
- *Yerba Buena* (mint)—used for colic; diarrhea; menstrual cramps; and intestinal influenza.
- *Ajo* (garlic)—used for decreasing arterial pressure; treating certain worm (parasitic) conditions; arteriosclerosis; and bronchitis.

DISLOCATION OF INTERNAL ORGANS

Aside from the types of illnesses already described, Mexican-American folk beliefs include still another category of diseases—dislocation of internal organs. The most prevalent such condition is *mollera caida* or fallen fontanel.

This condition is believed to be brought about by dropping or bouncing a baby too hard or by removing the nipple too roughly from the baby's mouth, thus causing the fontanel to sink and in turn make the palate bulge. This bulging interferes with the infant's eating. Symptoms include poor sucking at the breast or bottle, excessive crying, diarrhea, sunken eyes, vomiting, and sometimes fever.

Three different treatments in series may be used for *mollera caida*. First, a finger or thumb is inserted into the infant's mouth and the palate pushed gently upward, back into place. Second, the baby is held upside down over a pan of tepid water so that the tips of his hair barely touch the water and the soles of his feet are slapped one time. The third procedure is to apply warm salted olive oil to the fontanel depression. These procedures are generally performed separately on three consecutive days(3).

Of all the conditions listed thus far, this problem is most difficult for the health professional to handle. The cultural belief in the cause and treatment of the symptoms of *mollera caida* is very strong in each generation. Prompting the mother to seek medical attention as soon as possible and to accept medical intervention, including hospitalization, is often necessary. In too many cases when the mother finally does seek medical attention, the clinical symptoms of dehydration are already apparent.

Other folk illnesses involving dislocation of organs are *bolitas* (small lumps or masses in the tissue of the arms and legs) and barrenness in women, associated with a "fallen or twisted uterus." Treatment of both disorders involves massage or physical manipulation. In the case of barrenness the abdomen is massaged with oil until "the womb is put back into place"(4).

EMOTIONS AS A CAUSE OF DISEASE

A fourth group of diseases identified in Mexican-American beliefs are those connected with the experience of emotion. When an adult becomes extremely angry and explodes into an uncontrollable rage, for example, he is believed to be open to a condition called *bilis*. A day or two later he will suffer acute nervous tension, chronic fatigue, and malaise. The most striking symptom of *bilis* is yellow skin.

Many women attribute their newborn's jaundice to their own *bilis* during pregnancy. A simple yet thorough explanation of newborn hyperbilirubinemia may be helpful to both mother and father in accepting its treatment. Equally important is alleviating the mother's guilt, especially if she feels she may be to blame for this condition in her newborn.

Susto is another emotionally-based illness. *Susto,* or fright, is usually the result of a traumatic experience, which may be anything from witnessing an accident or death to a simple scare at night. *Espanto,* another form of *susto*, is thought to be caused by fright due to supernatural causes. In *espanto* the spirit leaves the body as a result of the scare.

Symptoms of these folk conditions are fretful sleep or insomnia, depression, apathy, and extreme tiredness. A *curandera* treats *espanto* by having the patient lie down on the floor with his arms outstretched in the position of a cross. Then sweeping his body with herbs and praying, she coaxes the lost spirit to re-enter the victim's body.

If simple *susto* is not recognized and treated immediately, it progresses to *susto pasado,* requiring an *ensalme* or blessing by a priest. Cases of *susto* which are permitted to progress, either through delay in treatment or through using a practitioner not equipped to handle such conditions (such as a doctor), are believed eventually to prove fatal(5). Thus, patients and their families may strongly resist referrals for professional help. Careful observance of continued depression and psychosis is therefore of paramount importance in caring for people of this culture.

Like emotions, blood is linked very closely to health and disease in the Mexican-American's system of beliefs. Blood loss, even in very minute amounts is thought to cause weakness and in males to impair sexual vigor. Furthermore, anemias are often associated with tuberculosis. Much teaching about diseases of the blood is therefore indicated.

A number of diseases identified in the folk medicine of Mexican-Americans do not fall in any particular category. *Empacho* is one such condition believed to be caused by a bolus of food sticking to the abdominal lining, causing swelling. Symptoms include lack of appetite, abdominal pain, slight diarrhea, vomiting, fever, restlessness, and—in children—crying. It is said to be diagnosed by feeling the calves of the legs for bundles of knots along the nerves. If such lumps are found in the calves, the abdomen is palpated and in *empacho* a large hard ball in the stomach may be felt(2).

The condition, attributed to excess intake of cheese and eggs (in infants only) and of bananas and soft bread is usually treated by a *curandera* or an older relative who has an understanding of the disease. The goal of treatment is to dislodge the bolus of food from the wall of the stomach. This is done by rubbing the stomach and by pinching and pulling up on the skin of the back in small folds at every third vertebra and then releasing it. This is repeated until three pops are heard, signifying the dislodgement of the *empacho*. Finally an herbal tea with some cathartic qualities is given to the patient to "clean out the stomach."

Adults strongly believe in routine use of cathartics to keep the stomach clean and prevent *empacho*. Their "overuse" of these preparations should be prevented by counseling them about dietary habits that produce the same effects as well as by stressing the dependency they may build up for laxatives if they use these drugs indiscriminately.

MISUNDERSTANDINGS OF STANDARD DISEASES

Aside from all the diseases included in their folk medicine, a fairly large group of standard, scientifically identified diseases are recognized by the Mexican-American people. Among a few are tuberculosis, cancer, pneumonia (*pulmonia*), asthma *(asma)*, measles *(sarampion)*, chicken pox (*virjuela loca*), polio, whooping cough (*tos ferina*), and diphtheria *(dipteria)*. Often, however, the etiology of these illnesses may be misunderstood and the disorder attributed to some of the previously mentioned folk categories. Many Mexican-American tuberculosis patients who have been followed through public health agencies, for example, attribute their disease to *mal aigre,* to hot/cold imbalance, or to an untreated cold, eventually leading to tuberculosis.

While the Mexican-American's ideas about the causes and treatments of disease are important to consider, so are his attitudes in general about health care. It is a strong cultural trait for this group, for example, to have close ties with the extended family. When a person is ill, many of these family members are therefore involved in deciding if indeed he is ill in the first place; the extent of the illness; and the treatment to be implemented and by whom.

Those practitioners considered first are people who are members of the community and regarded as specialists because they have learned more of the popular medical lore than most people. The *sabadorra,* whose specialty is handling fractures and bone disorders; the *partera* or midwife; and, of course, the *curandera-ro* are among these. But even these folk healers are consulted only after personal home remedies have failed.

With the rising cost of hospitalization, it has been observed that many new Mexican immigrants obtain prenatal care (a maximum of one to three visits through a private medical doctor) and then—if there have been no problems—employ the services of a *partera* when delivery is near.

The *curandera,* or general healer, is consulted by many people because she has known them intimately for years, speaks their language, and never dictates orders for care but makes suggestions, leaving the ultimate decision up to the patient and his family.

If people from this culture do seek help from outside their community, often chiropractors, naturopaths, and herbalists rather than medical doctors will be their first choice. Although these marginal practitioners may not speak Spanish, the Mexican-American finds that aside from being less expensive than the physician, they are more able to relate to them. They find these practitioners to have a better "bedside manner" and a more understanding acceptance of Mexican-American traditional beliefs and practices than physicians(2). Furthermore, the means of therapy of such practitioners are often similar to those of the Mexican-American culture—massage, manipulation, and herbal treatments.

BLENDING NEW WITH OLD

If health professionals wish to be successful in treating Mexican-Americans, they should keep a few considerations in mind. First, they need to remember that Mexican-Americans believe in the extended family and almost always prefer to consult family members regarding treatment, especially in cases of hospitalization or prolonged therapy, before making a decision. Assuming a dictating manner will only push the patient and his family away since final authority always rests with the immediate family in this culture. Therefore practitioners will succeed only in defeating their own purpose.

Another critical point to remember is that many Spanish-and Mexican-Americans are bilingual and should be approached cautiously. They may have a strong preference for speaking in the language with which they feel most comfortable. If a patient speaks Spanish only or prefers this language, a Spanish-speaking doctor or nurse should interview him. If none is available, specially trained bilingual aides are best. Much is lost or misinterpreted by untrained interpreters in health care settings.

Directions for medications or treatments should be explained in detail and as simply as possible, and Spanish literature might be used to reinforce these verbal instructions. Complex explanations or scientific definitions of diseases serve only to confuse.

Since Mexican-Americans see illness as a presence of symptoms and a state of temporary disability, diseases having no visible signs should be explained in terms of their preclinical signs whenever this is possible —for example, unhealing sores, persistent coughing, and excessive perspiration. The patient should also be reassured as to the disease's course and eventual outcome.

As with many other ethnic groups, modesty is of great concern. Measures to preserve privacy should be observed at all times, with care taken to expose as little of the body as possible during examinations and treatments. Sexual topics also are very uncomfortable to older Mexican-American women. They are generally very reluctant to touch the genitalia of any of their sons, regardless of age. If possible, the father should be involved in any care which requires such intimate contact.

Finally, open-mindedness and tolerance of cultural beliefs is extremely important. Conflicts with or repudiation of these beliefs by Anglo health care providers leads to fear, distrust, and eventual rejection of their services. Rather than openly deny the existence of folk illnesses and the effectiveness of traditional home remedies, the health care worker should try to incorporate them into the plan of care. It is not necessary to destroy a people's culture to improve their health and well-being(16).

REFERENCES

1. SAUNDERS, LYLE. The Spanish speaking people of the Southwest. IN *Cul-*

tural *Differences and Medical Care.* New York, Russell Sage Foundation, 1954.
2. CLARK, M. *Health in the Mexican-American Culture; A Community Study.* 2d ed. Berkeley, University of California Press, 1970, p. 173.
3. MARTINEZ, CERVANDO, AND MARTIN, H. W. Folk diseases among urban Mexican-Americans. *JAMA* 196:162, Apr. 11, 1966.
4. CLARK, *op.cit.,* p. 172.
5. RUBEL, A. J. Concepts of disease in Mexican-American culture. *Am. Anthrop.* 62:795-814, Oct. 1960.
6. JOHNSON, C. A. Nursing and Mexican-American folk medicine. *Nurs. Forum* 3(2):102-112, 1964.

From *Nursing Outlook* 23:755-759, Dec. 1975. Copyright © 1975. AJN Co.

No Shows: A Problem in Health Care

CAROL J. LINDSTROM

Broken clinic appointments are more than annoying; they mean some children aren't getting good care. In a small study, Mexican-American mothers explained why they didn't come to clinic—and why they did.

Any nurse who has worked in a publicly supported child health clinic is aware of, and frustrated by, broken appointments or "no shows"— mothers who make, or are given, appointments which they do not keep. This is a matter of concern to health professionals, not only because of the problems it creates for clinic personnel but, more important, because it represents inadequate health care for the children who do not come(1, 2).

Who are the ones not keeping their appointments? Why? The literature suggests that poor health care, little preventive care, and broken appointments are associated with ethnic minority status, low income, low educational level, low skill occupation, low social class, residence in a poverty area, and large families(1, 3, 4). Reasons for not seeking care have been attributed to cost, lack of transportation, lack of a baby sitter, and poor understanding of the value of preventive care(2, 5, 6).

Those who fail to keep appointments, however, have received con-

DR. LINDSTROM *(BSPHN, University of Minnesota; M.P.H., University of Michigan) earned her doctorate at Michigan State University. She is associate professor in the College of Nursing, University of Arizona, and works as a volunteer in a nursing clinic in the south end of Tucson, functioning as both public health nurse and interpreter. This paper is based on a speech given at the APHA convention in New Orleans in November 1974. The data discussed were drawn from a study supported by the Division of Nursing, DHEW, grant No. F04-NU27-183-04.*

siderably more attention in the literature than those who keep appointments. I therefore began to wonder: Who does keep appointments? And why? Some answers to this question, I thought, might provide information which would be helpful in working with those who did not keep appointments, and I therefore undertook a small study in this area.

THE SETTING

The setting for my study was a clinic in which I had worked regularly for the first year and a half of its operation—a county health department child health clinic in Lansing, Michigan. The clinic was located in a low-income neighborhood; well child care, treatment for common childhood illnesses, and referral to other sources of care were provided for children under five in families who did not have access to or who could not afford private care. Blacks, whites, and Mexican-Americans attended in approximately equal numbers, and attendance patterns were similar in all three groups.

An effort had been made to take care of some of the more common factors interfering with clinic attendance. Volunteers, for instance, were available to provide transportation for those who needed it and also to look after the children while the mother was otherwise occupied. In addition, and insofar as possible, the mothers and children saw the same doctor and nurse at each visit.

The staff hoped that such continuity and attention to transportation difficulties would help to reduce the number of broken appointments. Nevertheless, the patterns varied. Some mothers brought their children to the clinic consistently and according to schedule, whether the children were sick or well. Some mothers brought their children, sporadically, usually only when they were sick. Some, of course, never came at all. Over time, the nurses had found they could look at the appointment book and predict that "this mother will come because she always comes" and "this mother will come only if the children are sick."

I became particularly interested in the Mexican-American families. In addition to suffering from poverty and all of its concomitant problems and characteristics, these families had a cultural background different from the other two groups, as was reflected in the fact that they spoke Spanish. I therefore decided to concentrate on this group and, mindful of the cardinal rule of public health nursing to "start where the patient is," I tried to find out whether the attendance and nonattendance of these mothers might be a function of their poverty, of their ethnicity, or of both.

Accordingly, my study was directed toward determining what factors differentiated those Mexican-American mothers who attended the child health clinic consistently, those who attended sporadically, and those who never attended. I wanted to understand the Mexican-American families, both in the context of their culture and in their articulation with the Anglo health care system.

WAS CULTURE A FACTOR?

Family relationships among Mexican-Americans are strong, male dominated, and extended, ethnographers say. Women are socially isolated; their role is to stay at home and care for the home and family. Children are valued and loved; families are large. Privacy, personal relationships, and individual dignity are important. What a man *is* is more important than what he *does*.

Health and illness and attitudes toward them are integral parts of the social life in the Mexican-American culture. Folk medicine is integrated with and reinforced by other elements of the culture. Contact with Anglo medicine seems to be limited and largely negative. The majority of the population is part of the lower social class, most of them still speak Spanish, and acculturation to Anglo ways is slow(7, 8, 9).

All of these ethnographic studies were done in the Southwest, in rural or semirural areas, or in Mexican enclaves in urban areas. For several reasons, however, it did not seem wise to generalize from these studies to the Mexican-American group that I studied in Michigan, for the latter were a self-selected group. Over half of the men were born in Texas and migrated to Michigan because job opportunities were better. In general, the men are better educated and have higher incomes than the men in the areas of Texas which they left. In Lansing, there is no one area populated exclusively by Mexican-Americans. It seemed possible that these families who chose to settle in Lansing might be ready to adapt to or accept some Anglo ways.

To a greater or lesser degree, all of these families are exposed to Anglos and Anglo ways. Most of the men have a continuing exposure at their place of employment. The children go to primarily Anglo schools. Many of them have Anglo neighbors, However, to a very high degree, these families' lives are influenced by Mexican culture. They speak Spanish, eat Mexican foods, play Mexican music, participate in Mexican festivals, and return often to Texas or Mexico to visit family members.

Nevertheless, these women probably know more about the Anglo culture than Anglos know about the Mexican culture. In the child health clinic, the mothers are participating in the Anglo health care system; public health nurses see them in contact with and in the context of that system. However, the mothers live in both cultures and may participate in both systems.

FINDING ANSWERS

When I began working with Spanish-speaking families, I was frustrated by my inability to communicate with them. At the clinic, there was usually someone available to interpret for the professional and the mother but I was never completely satisfied with this, because I did not know if the interpreter's bilingual vocabulary was adequate to the task. I therefore took an intensive course in Spanish, both to be able to communicate with the families and to gain some understanding of how they viewed the world. This proved invaluable in my contacts with the families during the data collection process.

In addition to knowing the language, I needed a good background in Mexican-American culture. A study of ethnography provided me with a picture of their way of life, their values, and how health and illness fit into their perception of life and living. When I was ready to begin interviewing, I knew what specific aspects of family life, health, and illness I wanted to observe and learn more about.

Since no one had studied the perceptions and behavior of Mexican mothers regarding health and illness in their preschool children, or related their perceptions to their utilization of preventive care in the Anglo system, I developed an interview specifically for this study.

The sample was composed of ten families who attended the clinic consistently (good users), ten who attended sporadically (poor users), and ten who had never attended although they had access to the clinic (nonusers).

Since I planned to introduce myself as a public health nurse, I fully expected that I would provide some nursing service to the families. I could not in good conscience refuse if there was a need which I could help the family to meet. The nursing director concurred with my plan and agreed that I would function as an ex-officio staff nurse while conducting the study.

Before I began interviewing the mothers, I talked with two of the leaders in the Mexican community so that they would know what I planned to do. Both expressed interest in and approval of the study. They felt that I would be accepted into the homes readily because people respect public health nurses.

INFORMAL INTERVIEWS

This expectation was fulfilled; I was indeed accepted readily. I introduced myself by name as a public health nurse, and was always invited to come in. I then explained that I was doing a special study because I was particularly interested in Mexican families; I felt that public health nurses needed to know more about them in order to work well with them. I asked the mother if she would be willing to talk with me and answer some questions about herself and her children. Every mother whom I contacted agreed to participate.

I had at least two contacts with each family except one over a period of ten months. This enabled me to conduct the interview at a leisurely pace, follow clues for further information, and make some pertinent observations in the home, including family interactions. I had repeated contact over a period of months with three families in each group.

All of the mothers talked to me willingly and freely. The interviews were conducted informally, often at the kitchen table. They were delighted that I spoke some Spanish; we frequently used a mixture of Spanish and English. In twelve of the families, the father expressed interest in what I was doing and participated actively in the discussions.

In the good and poor user groups, the families in the sample were the first ten whom I visited in each group. As for the families who had never attended the clinic and were nonusers, I found some by accident, some through the families I knew, and some through the staff nurses.

I have no way of knowing whether the information given me by the mothers reflected their true feelings, beliefs, and behaviors. Neither do I have any indication that it did not. I assume the truth of their responses for several reasons. For one thing, they all had the option of not participating. For another, the mothers talked to me freely and at great length, and many of them volunteered information of a highly personal nature, which indicated acceptance and trust, I thought.

SIMILARITIES AND DIFFERENCES

The 30 families in this study all had low incomes; eleven families had an income below $5,000 and only two had an income of $10,000. Many had had little education; for instance, one father and five mothers had not attended school at all; six fathers and one mother had finished high school; none had gone beyond high school. The majority lived in poor neighborhoods, in deteriorating housing.

They shared a number of other characteristics. Family relationships were strong, male-dominated, and extended. Most of the women were socially isolated. They valued privacy; of the 26 families who had a phone, all but three had an unlisted number. Personal dignity was important; they did not like to ask for help.

There were some differences between them, however, and one difference between the good and poor users became apparent as soon as I started analyzing my data. In the group of good users, there were only three nuclear families—father, mother, and children of that union. By contrast, in the poor user group there were nine nuclear families.

Four of the women in the good user group were functioning as heads of household. Three of the women were married for the second time; each had children of the first marriage living with them. These seven women had in common a feeling of complete responsibility for their children—a responsibility which those without a husband in residence felt for all of the children and those with a husband felt for the children who were theirs but not their husbands'.

In this situation, these mothers were forced to assume more responsibility than the mother in a nuclear family. They seem to have responded by becoming more independent than the women in nuclear families. As one mother said, "When my husband died, I *had* to do things." This independence, coupled with increased responsibility in the care of their children, may account in part for their consistent use of child health clinic services. Since these mothers lack the support of a husband in the care of some or all of their children, they turn to other sources for help.

This family structure—being or having been head of a household—was a good predictor of good use of the clinic. Age, family size, and command of English were similar in all three groups. Average income was about $1,000 higher for the good user group. Education of the mother did not predict good use; the mothers in the poor user group were the best educated.

Place of education or, more broadly, socialization of the parents, particularly the mother, may be predictive. A number of parents said that Mexicans get a poor education in Texas. One young mother told me "Schools don't think Mexicans are important." In the good user group only four mothers and four fathers were educated in Texas, compared with seven mothers and six fathers in the poor user group.

The mothers who were socialized in Texas reported few contacts with the Anglo health care system there, and those were largely negative experiences. All said they could not afford medical care. A few knew about well child clinics but had never gone to one. Several said, "Clinics are for white people." (The people of Mexican heritage who participated in this study referred to themselves as "Mexican" and to light-skinned Caucasians as "white.")

PRENATAL AND CHILD CARE

Preventive health care for children apparently is related to the mother's use of prenatal care(10,11). Mothers in the good user group began prenatal care earlier than mothers in the other two groups. Only one mother had never had prenatal care. Of particular interest to me was the fact that nine mothers (three in each group) said they had had little, late, or no prenatal care in Texas, but that they had begun to have care early in their pregnancies in Lansing.

Since there is a relationship between use of prenatal care and use of preventive care for children, I asked the mothers why they had prenatal care. Only two mothers said they began care early and continued regularly because they were sick. One mother began early and went regularly "because it's what you're supposed to do." Another mother went because the doctor told her to. The rest of the mothers went because they thought it best to be sure they and the baby were all right. This suggests that they had an understanding of preventive care which might perhaps be extended to provide preventive care for their children.

All of the mothers in the good user group knew that they were bringing the children to the clinic for preventive care—"to be sure they are okay"—as well as for immunizations and treatment for some illnesses. One mother was glad she took her son regularly because one time she found out that his blood was "thin" and that "scared" her. They gave her some medicine and told her what he should eat. When she took him back, his blood was better; that made her feel good. Both good and poor users were consistent in returning for a check on a low hemoglobin; all but one of the children showed improvement.

Seven of the mothers in the poor user group had brought the children to "baby clinic" to see how they were. The other three mothers only wanted "shots" and thought they were going to an immunization clinic. Some of the mothers in the nonuser group also confused the child health clinic with the immunization clinic; they are held in the same place, but on different days.

WHY THEY BROKE APPOINTMENTS

The mothers gave various reasons for the broken appointments. Several did not think more check-ups were necessary, once they knew the child was all right. Several were overwhelmed with a large family and had all they could do to get to the doctor for illness.

Four mothers named lack of transportation as one or the only reason for not keeping appointments. I wondered about this because I knew that transportation was provided for mothers who needed it, but the nursing supervisor said that only the aggressive mothers will ask for such transportation. I checked the appointment sheets for 1972. Only seven of the 87 Spanish-surnamed families who had appointments had requested transportation. However, 14 of the women in this study reported that transportation was always or usually a problem. This illustrates the impression that these Mexican women are not very aggressive and do not like to ask for help.

One mother in the nonuser group knew about the clinic. The public health nurse had told her and she wanted to take her children, she said, but she did not have transportation. Three of the mothers in this group had had private preventive care for their children in the past, but now they could not afford it. Two of these mothers became good users during the course of the study. Predictably, one was and one had been the head of her household.

Five mothers in the nonuser group did not think it necessary to take a child to the doctor unless he is sick. One mother had gone to the child health clinic with her daughter-in-law to help with her two children. I asked if she had ever taken Rafael, her own four-year-old. She looked at me in surprise and said, "Oh, no. Why would I do that? Rafael is *healthy*. No need to take away time from children who aren't."

FOLK MEDICINE

All of the mothers valued good health for their children, did what they could to keep them healthy, and got upset and frightened when they got sick. All of the mothers treated sick children at home before seeking any outside help. Aspirin, Vicks, fluids, and observation were the most common responses to the question about home remedies. Treatment at home included folk treatment for folk diseases.

For example, *empacho,* a form of indigestion, results when a ball of undigested food gets stuck on the wall of the stomach or intestine. It causes pain, swelling and loss of appetite; the hard ball may be felt. It may be caused by eating a food which disagrees with one, or by eating too much. It may also be caused by eating food which one does not like or want to eat, or at a time when one does not want to eat. For example, if a guest eats food he does not want out of courtesy to the hostess, he may get *empacho.*

The mothers were surprised that I knew about Mexican folk diseases. I described them and asked each mother if any of her children had ever had any of these diseases or if she knew of children who had. If a mother knew of an occurence, this meant she believed in the folk system.

Three of the mothers said they did not know a great deal about the folk diseases. The remaining 27 knew a great deal about them, whether they believed in them or not. There was some difference in belief in the three groups. In the good user group, five women believed and five did not believe in the folk diseases. Eight mothers in the poor user group believed and two did not. Two of the eight named one disease in which they did not believe, however. In the nonuser group, seven mothers believed and one did not. Two said they "hardly believed"; they were beginning to wonder if the folk diseases were "real."

When a mother suspects that her child has a folk disease, she either treats him herself or takes him to a Mexican woman who can treat him. Folk treatment includes prayer, rituals, family involvement, and a great deal of tender loving care. A variety of herbal teas are used both for encouraging fluid intake and for their curative properties. Rice water is a fairly common treatment for diarrhea. One mother covered her child with wet leaves to reduce a fever. The folk remedies described to me are not harmful and many are helpful.

If the folk treatment does not work, the mother concludes that the child does not have a folk disease and takes him to the doctor. Thus, it can be seen that these mothers participate in two separate health care systems. Folk diseases are treated in the folk system; Anglo doctors do not know anything about them and cannot treat them. Nonfolk diseases are treated in the Anglo system.

When a child was sick, his mother was likely to seek medical care at the same point, whether or not she believed in the folk system. All of the mothers took the child to the doctor if what they did at home did not work or if they judged the child to be "really sick."

SUMMARY

The mothers who kept their appointments were likely to be or have been head of household; they had to assume more responsibility and independence than the mothers in nuclear families. They were more likely to have been socialized in Michigan or Mexico than in Texas. They were more likely to have transportation available. They brought their children to the clinic to be sure they were all right. They tended to have prenatal care early and regularly for the same reason.

The mothers who broke a number of appointments lived in nuclear families. They had never had to assume the total responsibility for their children. Unlike the good users, they were more likely to have been socialized in Texas. Some did not keep appointments because they did not have transportation. Some did not see any reason to take a child to the doctor unless he was sick. However, many of them did have prenatal care to be sure they were all right.

"Start where the patient is" is still a good precept for public health nursing practice. Understanding where these mothers are should enable us to adapt our approach and practice to help them achieve their goal of good health care for their children.

REFERENCES

1. ALPERT J. J. Broken appointments. *Pediatrics* 34:127-132, July 1964.

2. MORRIS, N. M., AND OTHERS. Deterrents to well child supervision. *Am. J. Public Health* 56:1232-1241, Aug. 1966.
3. HOCHSTIM, J. R., AND OTHERS. Poverty area under the microscope. *Am. J. Public Health* 58:1815-1827, Oct. 1968.
4. WINGERT, W. A., AND OTHERS. Demographical and ecological characteristics of a large urban pediatric outpatient population and implications for improving community pediatric care. *Am. J. Public Health* 58:859-876, May 1968.
5. PETERS, A. D. AND CHASE, C. L. Patterns of health care in infancy in a rural southern county. *Am. J. Public Health* 57:409-423, Mar. 1967.
6. GALLAGHER, E. B. Prenatal and infant health care in a medium-sized community. *Am. J. Public Health* 57:2127-2137, Dec. 1967.
7. CLARK, MARGARET. *Health in the Mexican-American Culture.* 2d ed. Los Angeles, University of California Press, 1970.
8. MADSEN, W. *Mexican Americans of South Texas.* 2d ed. New York, Holt, Rinehart and Winston, 1973.
9. RUBEL, A. J. *Across the Tracks.* Austin, University of Texas Press, 1966.
10. SCHOENFIELD, JACOB, AND OTHERS. Variations in prenatal care and well child supervision in a New England city. *J. Pediat.* 61:430-437, Sept. 1962.
11. SMILEY, JANE, AND OTHERS. Maternal and infant health and their associated factors in an inner city population. *Am. J. Public Health* 62:476-482, Apr. 1972.

From *Nursing Outlook* 25:320-329. May 1977. Copyright © 1977. AJN Co.

Healing Herbs, Gods, and Magic

Folk Health Beliefs Among Filipino-Americans

JOAN L. McKENZIE • **NOEL J. CHRISMAN**

Nursing care plans may be enriched by the incorporation of folk health practices, since some are biologically beneficial and all have significance for the cultural group.

Never go to bed with wet hair because you will go blind.

Boil corn hairs and water; drink and the urination will come out.

Do not let the fly step on your food. The witch has the power to send lice, flies, or cockroaches to you.

The above quotations are examples of Filipino-American folk health beliefs as expressed by Filipino-Americans themselves.* Like members of other American ethnic groups, many Filipinos continue to practice folk medicine because "it works." In some situations, folk remedies are their only treatments; in others, they combine folk remedies with the medical therapy prescribed by doctors and nurses. These folk beliefs are an important part of the people's daily lives and can significantly influence their experiences in the health care system.

Folk medicine has a long history—much longer than that of contemporary scientific medicine. Anthropologists attribute the persistence of folk beliefs to the fact that they are closely interwoven with other aspects

---

*Demographically varied, this group, interviewed by one of us (J.M.), included a 69-year-old-grandmother who is an artist and runs a handicraft business; 42-year-old mother of three children; 29-year-old woman currently obtaining a master's degree in social work; 32-year-old man attending college; 62-year-old grandmother, retired from teaching; 42-year-old nurse; retired registered nurse currently working as a volunteer; 40-year-old man employed as a medical technician; 42-year-old housewife and cosmetologist; and 58-year-old housewife employed as a machinist.

of a traditional society's life and culture. In addition, the therapeutic value of many of the health practices is verifiable scientifically(1).

The Filipinos' heritage is diversified. Based primarily upon Malayan culture, Filipino traditions have been influenced also by Indian, Chinese, Arabian, Spanish, Mexican, and American belief systems. Elements of health practices found in the Philippines today may have been borrowed from these cultures, particularly the Chinese(2).

Filipinos associate disease with the total life situation and with both natural and supernatural causation. Home remedies—herbal preparations, teas, and massage—as well as sleep and exercise are employed frequently for the treatment of illness attributed to natural causes such as overeating, poor diet, excessive drinking, physical abuse of the body, infections, and accidents. Many spices—for example, garlic, ginger, vinegar, and salt—are thought to have special powers, and the importance of touch is stressed.

SUPERNATURAL INTERVENTION

Belief in various supernatural causes of disease is widespread(3). The spirits of departed ancestors, witches, sorcerers, mediums, and nonpersons may all be seen as instrumental in bringing on illness or misfortune; environmental forces such as the wind, moon, and night air may also play a part. Individuals may be protected from harmful supernatural influences by talismans, amulets, and prayer, or resort to a folk healer, through whom they recruit assistance from the supernatural for divining future events, maintaining social relationships, ensuring success in personal matters and business, and curing the insane and the alcoholic. Although Western scientific practitioners are available and frequently used, most Filipinos recognize that these doctors are unable to cure supernaturally imposed illness.

When Filipinos move to the United States, they tend to transfer aspects of their homeland's folk belief systems to the new environment(4). Thus, Filipino-Americans blend the natural and the supernatural in their beliefs about health and illness in much the same way as native Filipinos. They have definite ideas about health and illness and have developed a

JOAN L. McKENZIE, R.N., M.N., *currently a nursing consultant in occupational health, Department of Social and Health Services, Washington State, was an instructor of family and community health nursing at the University of Washington School of Nursing at the time this article was written.* NOEL J. CHRISMAN, Ph.D., M.P.H., *is an assistant professor in the Department of Community Health Care Systems and advisor for the graduate program in cross-cultural nursing at the University of Washington.*

complex and consistent system for coping with disease. This is readily shown by some typical responses to questions about the causes of illness:

I don't know—maybe carelessness, cold in the winter. Coldness goes to the palms of your feet and before you know it you are sneezing and cold will develop into worse than that.

The wind in the body is disturbed and it causes a weak link that causes people to get sick.

One young woman said she was convinced that sickness is caused by evil spirits—sometimes by witches. A Filipino health professional, currently practicing in a local hospital, prefaced her explanation of illness with the remark, "I don't usually tell Americans about the old ways. They think you are nuts." But, she explained, the spirits *do* have something to do with illness. "If you really believe, then God can do it," she continued, "and the devil can do it the other way, too." One man said he believed that those who use herbs and plants instead of visiting a doctor will live longer.

Folk remedies endure on adopted soil because they are well known, accessible, and trusted; because they are relatively inexpensive; and, most important, because of their perceived success in solving everyday health matters. American health professionals, however, are not likely to be familiar with these traditional beliefs because they are rarely revealed to them. Ignorance about Filipino-American folk health practices, however, will not prevent the Filipino's use of them in solving health problems. He will often employ folk medicine both before and after consulting a scientific practitioner. For example, one father said:

Oldest girl is in the hospital, and the fever will not go down. Brought her home and the quackdoctor massage to her back. No more fever. It works.

The "quackdoctor" refers to a native healer or folk health practitioner. He is completely acceptable to the Filipinos, but they fully understand that scientific medicine does not accept his role. Having specialized knowledge of traditional cures, he is sought when Western health professionals, uncomfortable with healing herbs, gods, and magic, show lack of concern, are too slow to cure a patient, or fail to cure him.

UNDERLYING RATIONALE
Three concepts underlie Filipino-American health beliefs and prac-

tices—flushing, heating, and protection—with each one identifying a basic process used in promoting good health. Flushing keeps the body free from debris; heating maintains a balanced internal temperature; and protection guards the body from outside influences. Although Western scientific concepts are similar, Filipino theories are founded on different premises. Flushing is based on the notion that the body is a container which can collect impurities; heating ties in with the belief that hot and cold qualities must be balanced in the body; and protection involves safe-guarding the body's boundaries from supernatural as well as natural forces.

Flushing is not a mere recipe for purging the physical body. It is a complex system of stimulating perspiration, vomiting, flatus, or menstrual bleeding for the purpose of removing evil forces harbored in the body. Vinegar is commonly used for flushing the body in an attempt to cure a fever or chest cold. Water, salt, or hot peppers are sometimes mixed with the vinegar, but the result is usually the same: "It causes the person to perspire and removes all the bad things from the body."

Another method used in treating fever and colds is to fry fresh ginger and lemon in olive oil and have the patient drink this mixture, which will induce the expelling of phlegm. Whatever the remedy, implicit in the flushing concept is the need to allow some particular thing to get out of the sick body(5). For instance, the person with a bad cough rubs lemon on his back and chest both morning and night to "open his pores and let the cough out." Urine is released by drinking boiled corn hairs and water, and chicken pox "gets out" of the body by deferring a bath for a week. To rid the body of gas or a sour stomach, rice is burned in the oven and, while still hot, is plunged into cold water. The person then drinks the water while it is still sizzling.

Ritual may accompany the flushing in an effort to enhance the cure. For example, one mother says a little prayer while covering the "irritable stomach" with warm rice because she believes this gets rid of bad spirits. For the best results, herbal medicines are prepared only on special days and at certain times, such as on Good Friday at 12:00 noon(6).

Elaborate cleansing rules are carefully observed in the care of menstruating women and new mothers. Following delivery, a woman is confined to bed for two weeks, with the head of her bed slightly elevated in order that old blood and impurities may drain downward and out. A heavy menstrual flow is considered healthy because it removes "dirty" material from the system. In addition, reading and sewing are discouraged. When asked why new mothers should not read after giving birth, one woman stated:

That will never do. It will strain her eyes for even two months. Well, in childbearing everything is weak, they say, and I believe it because that is me now. I could hardly see. No, I did not believe it. I say that is only baloney. When I had my first child, I was still groggy from my anesthetic and yet my first request was to see the morning paper. So I read and I read. . . . I read so again with my second and third children. You know I cannot hardly see nothing now. I believe that—new mothers shouldn't read—now that it's too late.

THE POWER OF HEAT

Balance of hot and cold in the body plays a large part in Filipino-American health practices. An unhealthy body is thought to suffer from an excessive amount of heat or an invasion of cold. Too much heat, for example, will cause headaches. Some medicines such as camphorated oil and Sloan's ointment are viewed by Filipinos as hot, and the use of hot substances for curing is an important folk practice. Herbs, teas, water, and fire are often employed. For instance, ginger, considered to be a hot herb, is applied locally and used in conjunction with an elaborate system of massage in treating sprains, dislocations, torn ligaments, or sore muscles.

A sprain can also be massaged with hot peppers and oil, a practice believed to be useful because "heat goes there." For weakness, a tea of ginger and sugar is advocated since it will make the body warm. The same mixture can be sipped for a sore throat, cough, or hoarseness, because "it causes the throat to become very hot."

The role of heat in curing is aptly illustrated by the following example, which also provides a glimpse of how folk practices persist in the United States:

I have experience with my children just like a dream. When I come from the Philippines must call the doctor in the middle of the night. Doctor: "You do this and you do that and I come tomorrow." They do not come until after ten o'clock. I stand looking at my son perspiring, dying there, groaning. I cannot stand it so I pray to God and hope I could remember all the remedies my mother used to do us. My son he tremble like that. So I wrap him in a blanket, fill a bottle with hot water and then I roll that bottle on his body like that. That's how I stop him from wriggling all over.

Childbirth practices also include the use of heat. For example, a new mother is advised to sit in a special slotted chair over hot coals for one hour each day for nine days following delivery, to restore her reproductive organs. This procedure is called "drying" or "roasting." The woman is not allowed to bathe during the two weeks following birth or until the "fresh uterus" is returned to its normal shape and position. This is accomplished through the drying procedure and massages administered by a midwife. At the end of this time, a special bath is given that removes "dirty" substances from the body through perspiration. Until these procedures have been carried out to protect the "fresh uterus," the new mother is not allowed out of the house. She must also refrain from sexual activity for three months.

It should be noted, too, that heating and flushing are not discrete processes in the Filipino-American belief system; elements of both may be found in some health practices, as one older woman illustrates:

The urine is hard to go, so I sit in a tub of hot water as high as my waist with my head covered. I do it several times and I go and it really helps me. I wonder why doctors and nurses don't tell people this.

Protection provides a gatekeeping system against the invasion of both naturally and supernaturally imposed illness. The Filipino-Americans interviewed talked easily about evil spirits, witches, and dead ancestors, and it was evident that both Christian doctrine and magic were closely interwoven in their health practices. One woman explained that she was a Christian and knows that she shouldn't believe in evil spirits, but that she has been victimized by them. Another woman related that if a witch places a spell on someone, a coral stone or cross carried by the person will act as an antidote. When asked how one could recognize a witch, she answered that a witch "cannot stand your gaze."

As a matter of fact, the importance that Filipino-Americans place on maintaining eye contact has considerable implications for the delivery of health care services. If the nurse does not maintain eye contact, she could be perceived as the instrument of illness and misfortune—a witch—rather than a health care provider.

HELPFUL CURIOSITY

Nurses, unfortunately, tend to be uncomfortable with folk cures. But in order to promote therapeutic relationships with patients from different cultural backgrounds, it is necessary to become curious and knowledgeable about healing herbs, gods, and magic and plan interventions around cultural variations. When folk practices are clinically therapeutic or biomedically or psychosocially neutral, their integration into the nursing care plan will promote rapport with the patient and improve the likelihood that other nursing measures will be carried out. The nurse can also express to the client and his family a genuine and positive curiosity about their folk cures and perhaps disclose and discuss some of her own personal folk remedies.

Cures should not be shunned merely because they are expressed in culturally different terms or based on different cultural assumptions. Further, it is unwise to assume that folk remedies are harmful, since there are many successful applications of folk medicine. When a baby has colic, for example, the Filipino mother may rub her hands together until they are warm and then put them on the infant's abdomen to relieve gas. There is little difference between this practice and that of the public health nurse who suggests that the mother give her baby warm water and place the infant on his stomach to create a slight pressure. Likewise, there is nothing detrimental about flushing the feverish patient with fluids or prescribing ginger tea for a cold. In fact, ginger is a general stimulant that restores strength and has a carminative effect on the body. Ginger ale is used in many hospitals to provide patients with needed fluids and calories.

The folk treatment for sprains, dislocations, and sore muscles, geared to providing heat, involves massage and a ginger mixture. Nurses will immediately recognize the importance of massage and heat in speeding the healing process. By supporting the use of ginger along with common Western nursing interventions, nurses can increase the patient's acceptance of the treatment.

The blending of folk remedies with scientific cures can help bridge the communication gap between nurse, client, and family, thereby increasing trust. Once trust is established, the individual and his family will be much more open to the replacement of a potentially harmful folk practice by a medically validated one. Making fun of their beliefs and practices, as some nurses and physicians have been known to do, will keep clients from revealing them but not necessarily from practicing them. If a folk practitioner is significant to the patient and is willing to participate in his care, he should be included in the nursing care planning.

It is time for nurses to take the lead in recognizing the culturally pluralistic nature of American society. Consideration of the patient's point of view is an important aspect of the nursing process. Further, it may well be that folk health practices have therapeutic values as yet unknown to scientific researchers. In any case, open and sympathetic consideration of folk beliefs is likely to yield new and more acceptable nursing care plans for culturally distinctive persons.

REFERENCES
1. ACKERKNECHT, E. H. Natural diseases and rational treatment in primitive

medicine. *Bull. Hist. Med.* 19:(5):467-496, 1946.
2. HART, D. V. *Bisayan Filipino and Malayan Humoral Pathology: Folk Medicine and Ethnohistory in Southeast Asia.* Ithaca, N. Y., Cornell University, 1969. (Unpublished doctoral dissertation)
3. LIEBAN, R. W. *Cebuano Sorcery: Malign Magic in the Philippines.* Los Angeles, University of California Press, 1967.
4. MCKENZIE, JOAN. *A Descriptive Study of the Traditional Folk Medical Beliefs and Practices Among Selected Filipinos in Seattle.* Seattle, Washington, School of Nursing, University of Washington, 1974. (Unpublished master's thesis)
5. SNOW, L. F. Folk medical beliefs and their implications for the care of patients. *Ann. Intern. Med.* 81:82-96, July, 1974.
6. CLARK, MARGARET. *Health in the Mexican-American Culture; a Community Study.* 2d ed. Berkeley, Univ. of California Press, 1970.
7. LEININGER, MADELEINE. Witchcraft practices and psychocultural therapy with urban U. S. families. *Hum. Organ.* 32:73-83, Spring 1973.

From *Nursing Research* 26:53-56, Jan.-Feb. 1977. Copyright © 1977. AJN Co.

A Study of Illness Referral in a Spanish-Speaking Community

RITA L. AILINGER

In an anthropologic study of illness referral among Latin-American immigrants three phases were ascertained: First, there was extended use of self-treatment. Second, referrals were made to the social network, particularly to people from the same country of origin. Finally, referrals to the professional network were made to professionals with the same cultural heritage.

Illness referral systems utilized by ethnic groups remain an important concern of social scientists and health professionals. Knowledge about illness referral can aid the nurse in her assessment of factors which influence clients' decisions to seek preventive and therapeutic health services and can be used in planning and implementing nursing services.

Background of the Study. Friedson(1) and Zola(2) studied illness referral by interviewing patients as they came into clinics and found what influenced the person's decision to come to the clinic but no clues as to what other alternatives were used for treatment by individuals who did not reach the clinic. Kasl and Cobb viewed this as a serious omission in that two aspects of illness behavior, self-medication and the use of nonmedical functionaries, were omitted(3).

RITA L. AILINGER *(Boston College School of Nursing, Chestnut Hill, Massachusetts: Ph.D., Catholic University of America, Washington, D.C.) is assistant professor, Nursing Education Programs, School of Health Services, Johns Hopkins University, Baltimore, Maryland. This study was supported by a Predoctoral Nursing Research Fellowship (5 F04-NU-27, 271-02), U.S. Public Health Service.*

This article presents findings from a study designed to elucidate the illness-referral system utilized by families of Latin-American origin when faced with illness incidents in their homes. To understand the illness-referral system, it was necessary to study the larger system of health and illness which included knowledge, beliefs, attitudes, and practices(4). The illness-referral system was defined as the process of selecting a health-care alternative by an individual who perceived that he was ill. These selections were analyzed in the context of the sociocultural system which was defined as a system of elements which provided a framework for viewing social and cultural influences. It included activities of daily living, priorities related to values, economic goals, migration process, family relations, demographic characteristics, and the social network of the cooperative. An illness incident was defined as an occurrence of illness regardless of the number of consecutive days it continued. If the same illness occurred in one month at different times, it was regarded each time as an incident. The term, Latin-American families, was defined as those in which the parents were immigrants from Latin-American communities.

Mechanic reminded of the importance of studying illness referral from the cultural viewpoint:

. . . cultural patterns and typical ways of life give substance to the manner in which illness is perceived, expressed and reacted to. To some extent the cultural context defines that conditions are recognized, the causes to be attributed to them, and which persons have legitimate authority to assess and define such conditions. Similarly, cultural definitions influence the consequences of being defined as having a particular condition(5).

Despite distinct methodologies and study populations, previous studies reported a series of phases and events which individuals experience between the time they perceive symptoms and where they seek treatment. Investigations differed, however, in how they described the phases of the referral process.

Freidson described the lay and professional referral systems with which the person interacts when illness occurs(1). The lay-referral system he described is predicated on a patterned sequence of steps through which individuals pass. The steps constitute stages forming an opinion about the nature of the complaint and what to do about it. Freidson noted two cultural variables in the lay referral system: one is the congruence between the cultures of the client and the professional; the other, the number and cohesiveness of the lay consultants interspersed between the perception of sequence of steps through which individuals pass. It is important to note that in his model, Freidson's professional culture is equivalent to the modern medical culture while all other health practitioners are part of the lay referral system.

Polgar referred to a health action system in discussing "the procedures used by laymen and specialists to promote health, prevent sickness and remedy sickness"(6). He identified three phases through which a person passes in illness self-referral. The first is the self-addressed phase wherein the client and the health actor are the same person. In the second phase, the person solicits help from another or receives help from another without request; this is called the lay-health action phase and usually includes members of the client's immediate social group. In the third or professional phase, the client becomes the patient by seeking care from a health actor who is recognized as a specialist by the group. This specialist may be either a shaman or a professional health worker. An important distinction between the Freidson and Polgar models of illness referral is Freidson's use of the term professional to refer only to the modern medical culture while Polgar uses it to refer to anyone who is recognized as a specialist by the group seeking care.

Another approach to illness referral among ethnic groups was described by Weaver in his study of Spanish-Americans in New Mexico(7). He defined the illness referral system as "a sub-system of the medical system which includes all health actors and their expected and actual behavior in illness situations." His model includes five phases: 1) the self-addressed phase; 2) the kinship phase which includes health consultants from the immediate family and bilateral kindred; 3) the community phase which involves friends, neighbors, and other influential persons of the surrounding areas and sometimes overlaps with the kinship phase; 4) the folk specialist phase which includes the culturally recognized practitioners; 5) the urban professional phase which includes all those who provide scientific health services which originate outside the traditional village culture. Phases two, three, and four correspond to Polgar's lay health action phase.

Other investigators have looked at factors which influence the decision to seek medical aid. The relevance of these studies to the present one is obvious. For example, Zola in his well-known study on the decision to seek medical aid, found that a socially conditioned selective process may operate in the decision for medical treatment. Irish-Americans sought help only after receiving the approval of others; Italian-Americans sought aid when their symptoms interfered with social and personal relations. Americans of Anglo-Saxon origin sought help when the symptom interfered with certain vocational or physical activities(2).

Studies of health and illness among Spanish speakers in the United

States have concentrated on the Mexican-American(8), the Spanish-American(9), and Puerto Ricans(10). These reports focused on other health issues and only incidentally mentioned illness referral. One consistent factor noted in illness-referral behavior among these groups is the reliance on self-referral to a variety of persons in the lay world.

Thus, most authors tended to agree that a process takes place through which patients pass when they first perceive themselves to be ill through to their final mode of therapy. It is in how the process is defined that authors differed.

Given the lack of agreement on the referral process and the assumption that cultural and social factors play a significant role in shaping that process, this study sought to describe the illness-referral system of Latin-American immigrants in the sociocultural context of an ethnic cooperative.

Methodology. A combination of approaches including focused interviews, family health calendar (FHC) recording, and the traditional anthropologic approach of participant observation was used during the course of the study, from February 1972 through March 1973. The study population consisted of 19 Latin-American immigrant families living in a cooperative in a fringe, low-income suburb of an eastern metropolis. The cooperative consisted of 52 units, and over half the residents were of Latin-American heritage. All families who were willing participated in the study. The participants were from a variety of Latin-American countries, including Colombia, the Dominican Republic, El Salvador, Nicaragua, Paraguay, and Peru. All were employed and fell into social class positions four and five on the Hollingshead scale(11).

A prospective study in a cooperative was chosen for several reasons. First, as a self-contained unit it provided the opportunity to study a target population within the confines of their home environment. Second, other than the work by Cohen and Fernandez(12), there is limited information on the Spanish-speaking minority from Central and South America. The setting of an enclave with the majority of occupants from these regions afforded a unique population. Finally, the approach to study of illness referral in the home situation rather than a health agency allowed for inclusion of all treatment and referral modalities. The investigator obtained verbal permission from participants. She explained that the goal of the study was to learn about what happened in their daily lives which affected their health and to describe what they did when they became ill. The research was conducted in Spanish.

This report presents findings from the FHC. Each family recorded in the FHC illness which occurred during a selected month. A structured family health diary had been used in studies by Alpert et al.(13). Egeland[1] and Weidman[2] also used a structured family health calendar. For the purposes of this study, the calendar was modified to a semi-structured instrument and families were asked to record the name of the person ill, symptoms encountered, remedies used, and the person who suggested the therapy. Modifications in the instrument were made in order to improve the validity and reliability of the instrument for use with this cultural group. For example, in previous studies families were asked to record illness, based on a provided list. In this study patients were asked to describe the symptoms in their own words.

The validity of the instrument was checked by pretesting it with a Spanish-speaking population in Colombia. Another test of validity was that data on illness referral collected by the use of the FHC was similar to that found by means of participant observation.

Findings. *Illnesses and Symptoms Reported.* There were 99 persons living in the 19 households. In 89 percent of these homes, illness incidents were reported on the FHC during a one-month period; 62 incidents were recorded and the average per family was 3.7. Half the mothers and fathers, one-third of the children, and two-thirds of the other household members such as extended family or boarders reported symptoms of illness (see Table 1). In the Alpert et al. study 93 percent of the families had illnesses, slightly more than in this study(13). The same percentage of mothers were ill in both studies but fewer fathers (one-third) were ill in the Alpert et al. study. They found no symptoms were recorded for relatives living with the families, whereas in this study illness occurred in the majority of other household members. The most frequently reported symptoms were upper respiratory infections, gastrointestinal disturbances, and headaches. Mothers reported more headaches and gastrointestinal complaints, fathers reported respiratory and gastrointestinal problems, and children had more incidents of respiratory problems. Nine families reported at least one chronically ill member; these included six children, three fathers, one mother, and one grandmother. The chronic problems ranged in severity from allergies requiring no apparent change in activities of daily living to diabetes and a neurodegenerative disease requiring severe alterations in lifestyle.

Illness-Referral Patterns. When the Latin-American immigrant perceived himself to be ill, he usually self-treated without consultation (see

[1] Egeland, Dr. Janice. Hershey Medical Center, Hershey, Pennsylvania. 1973. personal communication.
[2] Weidman, Dr. Hazel. Department of Psychiatry, University of Miami Medical School, Miami, Florida. 1973, personal communication.

Table 1. Frequency and Distribution of Family Members (N = 99) Reporting Illness Incidents (N = 62)

NUMBERS	FAMILY MEMBERS							
	MOTHER		FATHER		CHILDREN		OTHER[1]	
	N	(%)	N	(%)	N	(%)	N	(%)
Total in study	19	(100)	16	(100)	46	(100)	18	(100)
Persons reporting illness	10	(50)	8	(50)	16	(33)	12	(60)
Incidents of illness	18	(29)	13	(21)	18	(29)	13	(21)

[1]Others in household, e.g., extended family members, boarders

Table 2. Referral, Remedy, and Illness Reported in the Family Health Calendar

REFERRAL	REMEDY/TREATMENT	TYPE OF ILLNESS
Self-treatment (60%)	Home and herbal remedies, nonprescription or prescription medicines	Headaches Headcolds Menstrual complaints
Social network (10%)	Home and herbal remedies, nonprescription medicines	Headcolds Muscular aches
Professional network (30%)	Prescription medicines	Chronic problems (e.g., rheumatism, allergies, skin, gastrointestinal)

Table 2). FHC respondents reported self-treatment over 60 percent of the time for maladies such as headaches, headcolds, and menstrual complaints. Treatments included home and herbal remedies, nonprescription medications, and perscription medications.

The second mode of illness referral was made within the social network. At this stage the person who perceived himself to be ill received a recommendation for treatment by someone in the social system. In the FHC reports, approximately ten percent of illnesses were referred to kin and friends. Friends who interacted socially, such as neighbors from the same country of origin, were most frequently a part of this social network referral.

Illness referrals to the professional network accounted for 30 percent of the reported incidents. These contacts were almost exclusively to Spanish-speaking physicians. In no cases were there reports of contacts to folk practitioners or nurses. Referrals to the professional network were primarily for children and adults with chronic problems such as rheumatism, allergies, skin problems, and gastrointestinal disturbances.

Discussion. An important finding of this study was that family members did not necessarily pass through each step of the illness-referral process. There seemed to be several routes which they took on their way to regaining health. In most cases they self-treated and went no further. In some instances, if the person was dissatisfied with self-treatment, he went to the social network and if not relieved of symptoms went on to the professional network. Others went directly to the social network or professional network without self-treatment. While some respondents were satisfied with the treatment they received at the professional stage, others shopped around or returned to self-treatment. The frequent use of self-treatment may be explained by several factors. Symptoms were interpreted as "treatable," thereby warranting self-treatment, or referral to the social or professional network was not convenient given the priorities of daily living. While the extensive use of self-treatment was primarily for minor problems in this population, the possibility exists that lay management of symptoms which may not appear critical because of a cultural interpretation may in fact be indicative of serious illness.

The fact that respondents continued to take their self-prescribed remedies suggests that traditional practices continue to be a viable source of therapy among Latin-American immigrant families. Several factors contributed to the continued utilization of such remedies. First, family members who visited the home country brought back the remedies. Second, a Latin-American food store in the neighborhood sold the herbs. Third, members of the ascending generation living in the household were more familiar with traditional therapies.

That the social network was utilized, particularly with respect to the friends from the same country of origin, reinforces the notion that national origin was an important bond of solidarity among the immigrants.

The use of a professional network primarily consisting of Spanish-speaking physicians suggests that language and culture were important considerations in the selection of an agent in the professional network. While there was a health center within one block of the enclave, the immigrants did not use the services because of the lack of Spanish-speaking personnel.

The findings in this study were similar to those reported by Weaver in that the urban client has an abbreviated referral system. However, it differed from Weaver's in one important aspect. No folk medicine specialists were contacted by the study group whereas Weaver pointed to their use by urban clients who failed to receive satisfaction at the professional level(7). The data supported Freidson's description of the referral structure in which the client may go directly from self-treatment to a physician. Nevertheless, Freidson discounted the use of a healer unless the client was desperate(1). In this study, the data indicated that self-treatment might include reliance on remedies of folk healers as a modification which is made by the immigrant to the new cultural context. Findings suggest the notion of a "distant healer" in that although the healer himself is not consulted, his remedies are employed and relied upon.

Limitations. The illness-referral system is a complex process which occurs in a variety of settings. Only observations by the investigator and reports by informants are included in this study. The instrument used in the study, the family health calendar, also had its limitations. Women often had difficulty in completing it on a daily basis, presumably because of other priorities. However, on weekly visits the investigator reviewed the FHC with the family, and reminded them to complete entries. Not all the women had completed primary school and were limited in writing skills. Based on this experience, the author would suggest that the use of the FHC be limited to those who have primary school education, that weekly contacts be made for the purpose of reviewing entries, and that the calendar be used in combination with other methods of data collection.

Another limitation of this study was the population which agreed to participate. Reasons why other families did not participate are unknown.

Because the research was limited to families in one setting, it cannot be known to what extent generalizations about similar families are possible. However, the intent of studying a small number of families in depth was to develop hypotheses which may be explored in future research. It is also important to identify characteristics of these families so that comparisons with other families can be made in future research.

REFERENCES

1. FREIDSON, ELIOT. *Patients' Views of Medical Practice.* New York, Russell Sage Foundation, 1961.
2. ZOLA I. K. Culture and symptoms—an analysis of patients' presenting complaints. *Am Social Rev* 31:615-630, Oct. 1966.
3. KASL, S. V., AND COBB, SIDNEY. Health behavior, illness behavior, and sick role behavior, Part 1. *Arch Environ Health* 12:246-266, Feb. 1966.
4. AILINGER, R. L. *Illness Referral System of Latin-American Immigrant Families,* Washington, D. C., Catholic University of America, 1974. (Unpublished doctoral dissertation)
5. MECHANIC, DAVID. *Medical Sociology,* New York, The Free Press, 1968, p.52.
6. POLGAR, STEVEN. Health action in cross-cultural perspective. IN *Hand-*

book of *Medical Sociology,* ed. by H. E. Freeman and others, Englewood Cliffs, N. J., Prentice-Hall, 1963, pp. 397-401.

7. WEAVER, THOMAS. Use of hypothetical situations in a study of Spanish American illness referral systems, *Hum Organ* 29:140-154, Summer 1970.

8. CLARK, MARGARET. *Health in the Mexican-American Culture,* 2d ed. Berkeley, University of California Press, 1970.

9. SAUNDERS, LYLE. Healing ways in the Spanish Southwest. IN *Patients, Physicians and Illness,* ed. by Gartly Jaco, Glencoe, Ill., Free Press, 1958, pp. 189-206.

10. PADILLA, ELENA. *Up From Puerto Rico,* New York, Columbia University Press, 1958.

11. HOLLINGSHEAD, A. B. *Two Factor Index of Social Position.* New Haven, The Author, 1957. (Mimeograph)

12. COHEN, L. M. AND FERNANDEZ, C. L. Ethnic identity and psychocultural adaptation of Spanish-speaking families. *Child Welfare* 53:413-421. July 1974.

13. ALPERT, J. AND OTHERS. A month of illness and health care among low-income families. *Public Health Rep* 82:705-713, Aug. 1967.

Section III Nursing in Community Health Agencies

The articles in this section focus on innovative practices in community health agencies. The first discusses an internship program one Visiting Nurse Association established to introduce new graduates to the complexities of nursing practice in the community setting. The next three articles describe methods for assessing the quality of care delivered by such agencies. Finally, a unique solution to the problem of developing and maintaining health record systems is presented, and the problem of protection for nurses working in potentially hazardous environments is explored.

From *Nursing Outlook* 23:374-377, June 1975. Copyright © 1975. AJN Co.

An Internship in Community Health Nursing

NORMA ACKERMAN • SUZANNE BAISEL

One response to the well documented theory-practice gap is the new internship program at the Boston Visiting Nurse Association, reported here.

What is a new baccalaureate graduate to do if she wants to begin her nursing practice in the community setting but the agency she would like to work for requires previous experience as a condition of employment? If that agency is the Visiting Nurse Association of Boston, she is fortunate, for this VNA offers the new graduate an alternative to previous experience—its own unique work-study program in community health nursing. The internship program was designed to prepare the beginning practitioner with effective and satisfying skills in community health nursing.

The VNA of Boston had come to realize that the increasingly complex demands of nursing in the community require skillful judgments and interventions in a wide variety of situations. To prepare new nurses to meet this challenge, the nine-month program was instituted in the fall of 1973 to bridge the gap from student to professional by means of a guided work experience.

THE FIRST INTERNS

We were the first interns to participate in the new program. Assigned to a district unit, we were responsible to its supervisory staff and were guided by a preceptor and the district supervisors through a predetermined schedule of progressive work experiences. We were responsible,

MISS ACKERMAN *and* MISS BAISEL *both graduated from the University of Michigan School of Nursing, Ann Arbor, and took part in the internship program at the Boston VNA described here.*

too, for independent study to supplement our clinical experience. Our preceptor for this experience was a master's-prepared community health nurse clinician whose background included both teaching and nursing service.

The program emphasis was on family and community health, and communication skills. During our nine months of internship, we were expected to make accurate and comprehensive nursing assessments and nursing diagnoses of families who had a wide variety of health and social needs. We were to provide nursing care, including therapuetic care, health counseling, and coordination of services. And we would evaluate the outcomes in light of family-patient progress.

Special attention was also paid to community health—becoming aware of the nursing needs of the community and collaborating with others in establishing diagnoses. Finally, developing new forms of communication in the community was stressed. We were expected to seek out opportunities to participate with consumers and providers in planning action groups.

As we began our internship we functioned as regular staff members, but with less than a full caseload of selected families. We gradually increased the number until, before the end of the internship, we were carrying a full average load. Each week the interns and the preceptor met as a group for two hours to discuss pertinent issues raised by either the interns or the preceptor. We occasionally used this time for observational experience in the community.

Also on a weekly basis individual conferences with the preceptor provided the opportunity to evaluate our progress or to pursue individual concerns. Our progress was evaluated periodically by joint assessment.

FAMILY HEALTH FOCUS

The weekly conferences with the preceptor proved to be a valuable learning experience for developing a family health focus. We discussed our assessments and plans and drew on the preceptor's experience to develop alternative approaches, set priorities, and identify appropriate community resources. The ongoing discussion of nursing intervention and evaluation of patient progress accelerated our growing competence.

The close collaboration between the preceptor and supervisory staff made possible a greater variety in the caseload assigned to the intern. It might include, for instance, a patient with cystic fibrosis, one with a complex ostomy problem, a terminally ill patient, a high-risk pregnancy, and a multiproblem family crisis. Occasionally, a visit was made by the intern and the preceptor together to evaluate the intervention skills further.

Initially, our weekly conferences focused on nursing assessment, nursing diagnosis, and recording techniques. Using supplemental reading and case examples, we discussed care of the elderly, the grief process, approaches to crisis intervention, high-risk pregnancy, effective involvement with the multiproblem family, and primary care nursing in community health. Some of our discussion topics aroused the interest of the entire district staff and resulted in staff education conferences.

From the beginning an awareness and knowledge of the community and its needs were an important part of our internship. The VNA provides home visiting for the federally funded maternity and infant care and child and youth programs, and field trips to these two clinics were helpful to us. More effective referral was made possible by contacts with the family planning clinic, the local mental health center, and a local planning and action center.

From attending the meetings of the community inter-agency council, we learned about other agencies and their services to the community. A day-care program for children of potentially abusive parents provided the opportunity for a first-hand look at the problem of child abuse. During our own district staff conference, we shared what we had learned and observed as we went along, so that all staff nurses could benefit from our outreach experience.

RESPONSIBILITY FOR INVOLVEMENT

As we began to learn about the community, we became increasingly aware of our responsibility to become involved in it. As a result, one of us worked to improve communication between the district visiting nurses and school nurses. She arranged a conference with the school nurses to discuss their role in the school and community. Later, at a joint conference, the district staff and school nurses discussed ways to promote better communication and collaboration in services to families they both served.

One of us concentrated on work with the elderly. A drop-in center for the elderly had recently been established by community organizers interested in the affairs of older persons, and we provided the nursing component by our participation one afternoon a week.

A little later, we initiated two blood pressure screening sessions at the center. Before long, the entire district staff was drawn into the work of this project to help handle the overwhelming community response. Data were tabulated and revealed that a significant number of the participants had been referred for medical care. The report indicated a need for further evaluation and possibly setting up a service to provide more frequent screening and follow-up.

The increase in size and activities of the drop-in center has resulted in more casefinding by the nurse and the establishment by the community of a hot-meal program at the center.

Our community involvement proved beneficial not only to us, we believe, but to the district staff and entire agency as well.

COMMUNICATION SKILLS

Developing skills in communication and collaboration had been identified as an important aspect of our learning. Our skills in these areas were broadened by organization of and participation in conferences involving clients and other professionals. Early in our internship, we participated in the VNA's coordinated home care program, which proved to be a good introduction to this area of learning. We were helped by the preceptor in arranging case conferences, making referrals to other agencies, and making use of the agency consultants.

We also paid attention to learning about the structure of our agency. Although it is large, before long we became aware of effective ways to initiate ideas. One such method was participation on agency committees. The internship allowed us to take advantage of this means earlier than we would have otherwise been able to.

One of us joined a cardiac task force that was already in progress and participated in the planning and carrying out of a project for better cardiac screening of families. She later became district representative to the staff council, in which staff members can voice their concerns and make recommendations to the administration.

She also became active with the legislative committee, which consisted of staff, administration, and board members, which reviewed legislation concerning home care agencies and provided information and recommendations based on their findings.

One of us devoted her efforts to the problem-oriented task force, which was established to design and implement a problem-oriented record system for the agency.

OUR REACTIONS

Our internship program was for us an exciting and stimulating experience in community health nursing. We chose it because it offered individualized attention and added learning opportunities. We truly made the right decision.

The individual conferences were an excellent opportunity to receive feedback. Discussing and analyzing our nursing care decreased the pressures of a new work experience and gave us valuable support. Having someone to listen to us and share with us, through those first months, helped build our self-confidence as professionals and increased our ability to function effectively. Joint home visits were an added learning opportunity.

With an increased feeling of security we were able to be more aggressive in our nursing care, setting up conferences, and communicating with other professionals.

Getting to know the community and becoming involved in its activities followed from our growing awareness of the community and from our own sense of responsibility. The program also provided a stimulus to self-evaluation and goal direction in our work. Periodic evaluation promoted an assurance that we were growing as professionals.

Due to the good communication and effective working relationships with our preceptor, only minor frustrations arose. One topic discussed and resolved was the amount of group conference time which could be used for field trips and community experiences within the agency framework. Program modifications were made with the preceptor to meet our individual needs and assure our continuing motivation and progress.

The internship program had been established to run for nine months. However, after six months we had gained a good understanding of our goals and of the necessary future experiences needed to achieve them.

After reviewing our achievement with our preceptor, we submitted an evaluation of our progress and an assessment of the program to the agency's administrative staff. We were then promoted to the level of Community Health Nurse I. We thus completed the internship with a feeling of increased responsibility to pursue professional goals.

EVALUATING THE PROGRAM

In making an overall evaluation of the internship program, the agency was able to draw upon the experiences of four baccalaureate-prepared staff members who had joined the staff without previous experience before the internship program had been introduced. Although no control group had been planned when the program was begun, these four staff members proved to be helpful in assessing the program's value.

In comparing the experiences of the interns with those of staff members, attention was given to the different levels of functioning of the two groups, the satisfactions and dissatisfactions that were felt, and the kinds of guidance and assistance that were provided.

The staff members who had not served an internship reported feelings of anxiety and turmoil during the first six months. They felt they had needed more "guided experiences." Freedom and independence in the community health nursing role did not provide a structure, and they had felt overwhelmed.

In contrast, the internship program had provided support and guidance. It had included the opportunity for a joint assessment of needs, the establishment of professional goals with periodic review of progress and reassessment, a structured plan with time allotments for getting to know the community and its services, guided experiences in analysis of the nursing process, pertinent field supervision for identified family problems, and continuing feedback about the intern's progress.

The internship proved to be advantageous for the agency as well as for us. It produced confident, well-prepared staff members six months after the new graduate began work. Actual monetary cost to the agency was computed on a cost-time analysis, with consideration of the time invested by the preceptor and the interns. Our salary rate as community health nurse interns was about $1,400 less than the beginning salary of the experienced nurse. However, upon completion of the internship, we then progressed to the salary level of the nurse with a year's experience.

THE FUTURE

With completion of the first internship program, the VNA of Boston has now made its internship program a requirement for all new baccalaureate graduates.

Five interns joined us in July 1974, and four more began in September. We assisted in bringing the agency staff up to date on the program in those districts where interns were to be assigned.

To handle the increased number of interns, additional preceptors have been appointed. They now include a community health nurse clinician, clinical assistants, and a senior staff nurse in addition to the original preceptor, who continues in charge of the program and participates in the weekly group conferences. This revised structure will be evaluated by the interns and preceptors upon completion of their program.

Besides its implications for new baccalaureate graduates, the internship has raised questions about any staff nurse entering community health. Many issues relative to the helping process are not unique to internship but warrant consideration for any new staff member. Certainly, of greatest benefit to the agency is the nurturing of professional confidence, expertise, and satisfaction in community health nursing, all of which increase the ability of the individual and the agency to give better service in delivery of health care.

From *Nursing Outlook* 25:168-171, Mar. 1977. Copyright © 1977. AJN Co.

A System To Evaluate Home Health Care Services

ELIZABETH A. DAUBERT

In an effort to assure and validate quality of care, this VNA developed a patient care review program in which records are assessed on the basis of specifically defined criteria.

Home health agencies claim that their services meet a basic community need and that the quality of care they provide is of high caliber. Such statements paint a picture of a multi-service delivery system of unquestionable worth that functions in an appropriate, adequate, efficient, effective, and clinically competent manner. When evidence is sought to validate such statements, however, it soon becomes apparent that little hard data exist to substantiate such glowing claims.

In reality, most evaluations of community health nursing and other agency service components are based upon individual assumptions and preferences, not upon substantive evidence. One reason might be the absence of a satisfactory method of measuring the quality of care provided, not only by nursing but by each of the other services offered by a home health agency.

There are, of course, some audit tools available; however, all have limitations. They either restrict themselves solely to an assessment of nursing or, if they have the capacity to appraise several services, their criteria are broad and not well defined. Without an operational definition of quality, or agreement about what constitutes "goodness" for each criterion of care, reviewers' judgments are guided by how they themselves would have given the care.

ELIZABETH DAUBERT, R.N., M.P.H., *is associate director of the Visiting Nurse Association of New Haven, Inc., Conn., and has held a variety of positions in community health nursing. This article is an expanded version of a speech presented at the American Public Health Association's annual Convention, held in Miami, October 1976.*

One possible solution to this problem is a method of quality assurance in the form of a patient care review program that has been developed by our visiting nurse association and has now been in operation for 18 months.

CHARACTERISTICS OF SYSTEM

The purpose of the review program is to provide a mechanism that will enable a systematic evaluation of the quality of patient care provided to individuals in their homes, in relation to (1) patients' needs due to illness or disability, and (2) the program objectives of the agency. The ultimate objective of the review system is to improve the quality of care by assisting the agency to provide a range of home health services at optimum standards. The review program's main characteristics are:

• It is a systematic appraisal of all home health services rendered by the agency, as documented in patients' records according to the extent to which these services measure up to the operational definition of quality care. This definition is derived from the standards of care as stated in the written policies of the agency.

• It has the capacity to assess the care provided by six disciplines—nursing, home health aide, social work, and physical, speech, and occupational therapy services.

• It is accomplished through the review of a statistically valid sample of active and discharged patients' records on a bimonthly basis to determine the extent to which 28 explicit care criteria have been met.

• It focuses on overall agency performance and measures those aspects of care considered essential in providing an integrated home health service of high quality. The degree of clinical competence of individual staff personnel is not directly evaluated; instead, an indirect assessment of staff performance emerges as a by-product of the review process.

• Finally, in these days of demands for accountability, the system is a tool to answer the question: "Does a patient receive good care?"

HOW THE SYSTEM WORKS

The process of record review is carried out by a group known as the Patient Care Review Committee, consisting of four experienced staff nurses, an administrator, and one nursing supervisor. During every review sequence, each committee member audits six or seven patient records. (No member is assigned a record of a patient in whose care she has participated.) The individual reviewers then present the findings of each record assessed to the total review committee for a final determination of the quality of service rendered, as well as for decisions regarding recommendations for follow-up.

A review form is completed for each record selected for audit. The form is divided into five sections designed to assess three dimensions of care: admission to service, delivery of service, and discharge from service. The first section, *Identifying Data,* is completed by a clerk and consists of basic information such as diagnosis, length of service, referral source, types and volume of services, and patient status, either active or discharged, at the time of review.

The next three sections are completed by the individual reviewers. The heart of the review is the second section, *Delivery of Services,* which consists of the largest number of items to be evaluated—such items as the care plan, visit schedule, physician orders, medication list, and the patient profile. Criteria for each item are described and defined in the instruction sheet, and the assessment is made on the basis of actual evidence in a patient's record that the criterion has been met. Thus, for "visit schedule," the description reads as follows:

As long as service is provided, the record shows that the visit frequency was safe and appropriate and that action plans were carried out as needed during each visit. Visit frequency should be consistent with M.D. orders and patient/family needs and should reflect any changes thereof. Long periods between visits (e.g., more than two weeks) which do not seem appropriate to the patient's condition should be explained in the narrative clearly (e.g., patient cancelled visit).

All reviewers, as well as the rest of the staff, have a copy of these criteria.

Each item on the review form is followed by spaces in which the reviewer checks "yes," "no," "uncertain," or "not applicable," according to whether or not the criterion has been met. "No" and "uncertain" answers must be explained in the space provided under "comments." The form for this section appears on page 120 and includes titles of items to be audited.

The same procedure is followed for the items listed in the third section, *Discharge from Service,* which is concerned with the reason for discharge and the patient's status on discharge, plans for discharge, and timeliness of the decision. In the fourth section, the *Primary Reviewer's Summary,* the reviewer summarizes the findings by entering the total number of criteria judged to be "yes," "no," "uncertain," "not applicable." In addition, the reviewer lists each item number that received a score of no or uncertain and the reason for the score.

The patient's record and reviewer's audit form then go to the total committee whose task is to judge the quality of the care on a 4-point scale from excellent (A) to poor (D). Guidelines defining criteria for each score

AUDIT SECTION II—DELIVERY OF SERVICES

	Yes	No	Unc.	N/A	Comments
12. M.D. Orders					
13. Medication List					
14. Housing					
15. Availability of Family/Friends					
16. Care Plan A. Medical Supervision					
B. Health Needs/Action Plan					
C. Referrals					
D. Safety					
E. Goals					
17. Patient Profile					
18. Communication with M.D.					
19. Visit Schedule					
20. Service Record					
21. Ongoing Care Plan A. Periodic Patient Assessment					
B. Periodic Alteration of Care Plan					
22. Involvement of Patient/Family					
23. Non-Nursing V.N.A. Services A. M.D. Orders					
B. P.T.					
C. H.H.A.					
D. H.H.A. Supervision					
E. Social Work					
24. Communication Between Nursing & P.T.					
Summary Admission to Service Enter Total Each Column					

Section II of the Five-Section Audit Form

are also included in the policy manual. For example, a score of excellent means no major defects were found or no more than two minor defects; for this score, no deficiencies can be present in the items identified as the care plan, visit schedule, ongoing care plan, physician orders, or any item under discharge from service.

Appropriate comments for the reasons for the scores are also recorded, as well as the committee's recommendation for follow-up actions, if indicated. These recommendations may be directed to the services being provided, agency policy, or coordination between community agencies, for instance. If some action is recommended, the committee specifies to whom the recommendation should be referred.

Following each record review sequence, a random sample of records rated excellent, good, fair, and poor by the review committee are reaudited and judged a second time by an impartial nurse. This monitoring mechanism assures accuracy and uniformity during the individual assessments by each reviewer as well as during the final deliberations of the review committee, in order to minimize the possibility of reviewer bias.

TESTING AND REVISION

During the testing phase of the system, the review form had 47 criteria to be assessed in the two main sections—delivery of care and discharge. After six months of use, the form was revised and the number of criteria reduced to 28. Some criteria were deleted because: (1) they were found to be purely mechanical indicators that evaluated the degree of adherence to the agency's record system, rather than the quality of services provided; (2) a few items never showed a deficiency; therefore, it was pointless as well as time consuming to continue assessing these items; and (3) two criteria dealt with team nursing, which no longer was practiced at our VNA; we had changed to district assignments. In some other instances, a few criteria were combined.

The revision of the form had two positive effects. First, it emphasized a more in-depth examination of the actual delivery of service and, second, the total time needed to complete the review form was reduced significantly, leading to a more effective, efficient patient care assessment tool.

The findings of each bimonthly review sequence are disseminated to all levels of agency personnel. For instance, each record requiring corrective action is returned to a supervisor who, in turn, discusses the review findings and the need for follow-up with the appropriate staff members. Once the corrective action has been taken, the supervisor responsible for monitoring the management of patient care notifies the review committee that the recommendations have been implemented.

Also following each review sequence, a written summary of all of the findings and recommendations is distributed to each service unit. Besides direct, formal feedback, periodic discussions concerning the findings and recommendations are held during administrative-supervisory meetings.

BUILT-IN BONUSES

This patient care review program has generated much new and worthwhile information. For the first time, hard data exist to document the quality of care provided by the agency. Also, statistics have been gathered concerning the average length of service required by certain types of patients and the volume and mix of personnel needed to provide appropriate care for each patient.

The program has also helped to identify agency strengths and weaknesses. Among the strengths identified were: responses to requests for service were promptly handled, physician orders were current and adequately executed, informal record reviews were done on schedule, on-site supervision of home health aides occurred regularly, and the skills of licensed practical nurses were appropriately utilized. A common thread ran through all of the identified strengths—that is, each strength could be classified as functional, or task-oriented.

WEAKNESS IDENTIFIED

The weaknesses that were uncovered ranged from too casual recording practices to inadequate development and execution of care plans. These, too, had a common trait; all weaknesses were in the knowledge-judgment area. For instance, some common deficiencies were incomplete listing of health needs and action plans as well as sketchy patient profiles, especially in the areas of secondary diagnoses and past health history. Other weaknesses were lack of involvement of family members in patients' care, timeliness of discharge, and adequacy of discharge planning. For instance, a patient would have been discharged to a hospital or nursing home but no evidence was found in the record to indicate that pertinent health or social data were relayed by the staff member responsible for the patient's care to the facility by phone or written summary.

To reduce the incidence of deficiencies and thus improve the quality of care, various kinds of remedial programs were undertaken. For example, staff education sessions were held to improve recording techniques, to increase knowledge concerning certain disease processes, and to develop skills in assessment and comprehensive care planning. In addition, changes were made in the agency's record system, and greater emphasis was placed upon adherence to established recording practices by all staff.

The test of any quality assurance program is its impact on patient care, especially its ultimate effect in dealing with the areas identified as problems or deficiencies. Recent review sequences have shown a significant improvement in the rating scores, demonstrating that the system has improved the quality of care. Furthermore, the list of common deficiencies has decreased from 13 to 3, which represents a 77 percent reduction.

Even though staff members were involved in the development of the system and inservice programs were held prior to its implementation, reaction to the process and its findings was mixed. Many staff members supported the concepts of quality assurance and accepted the fact that health professionals operate under a social mandate that expects them to be accountable for the quality of services rendered. Other staff members, however, appeared to neither accept nor support the concepts of quality assurance. Unfortunately, the system produced feelings of threat and rejection among the noncommitteed individuals.

How expensive is this program? Analysis has shown that it costs $590 to complete each review sequence. At the same time, the annual cost of the system, spread across the total illness service visits (59,566) made by our six illness service disciplines, is $.058 or not quite six cents a visit. Included in the cost are all salary and fringe benefits, time consumed completing individual record reviews and review committee meetings, preparation of committee minutes and reports, as well as time spent completing follow-up on records that were returned for corrections or recommended action.

FUTURE DIRECTIONS

At present, the system is working well and does answer the question, "Does a patient receive good care?" However, a second question—one equally important for home health agencies—needs to be addressed: "What difference does agency service make to a patient?" To find out, future efforts will be focused upon adding outcome criteria to the review procedure. By so doing, the system will then become a process-outcome method of evaluation. Continuing effort will be directed toward increasing the specificity of the rating scores.

Finally, a third modification is planned which will add another dimension to the system. Now, the primary reviewers also function as the total review committee but, in the future, the members will only assess individual records and complete the review forms. The final determination of the quality of care and recommendations for follow-up will be made by a committee composed of a physician, a nurse supervisor, two staff nurses—who are also primary reviewers—an administrator, a rehabilitation therapist, and a social worker. Such committee expansion should produce a multidisciplinary approach.

The system is not a finished product, but we believe that the valuable information we have already obtained has directly helped our staff to improve patient care and to make our services more responsive to patient needs. The fact that further refinement of our tool is necessary only serves to underline a fact that we all know: the search for an instrument to measure quality of care is a long and arduous task.

From the *American Journal of Nursing* 75:618-619, Apr. 1975. Copyright © 1975. AJN Co.

Peer Review in a Health Department

KARIN J. JOHNSON • MARY ANN ZIMMERMAN

As part of the annual evaluation, nurses and others in nursing service in Multnomah County, Oregon, assess their peers' working relationships and leadership potential.

Peer review does not start overnight. Community health nurses in Multnomah County, Oregon, found that it takes much time, work, and patience.

Our peer review started for two reasons. First, with the introduction of team nursing, job descriptions were rewritten, and nurses found that evaluation methods were too subjective. Second, the nurses began salary bargaining with the county commissioners, who challenged us to develop a system of evaluating professional performance.

The bargaining in 1971 was the first major attempt on the part of nurses to change the money structure of the department. Nonsupervisory nurses were classified in only two positions, community health nurse I and II. A nurse in CHN II had no option for advancement but to become a supervisor. At our salary structure, it was hard to attract and keep nurses for upper levels, so the bargaining team proposed a third level, CHN III, and merit, step-raises for CHN II and CHN III positions. CHN III was to be a position for staff nurses who were specialists in community planning or leadership. This would allow a nurse to be rewarded for excellence without being promoted to supervisor.

MS. JOHNSON, R.N., B.S., *was a nurse (CHN II) in the Multnomah County Division of Health Services, Portland, Ore. She is now a staff nurse at the Veterans Administration Hospital, Portland, Ore.* MS. ZIMMERMAN, R.N., B.S., *is a community health nurse and a pediatric nurse practitioner in the Multnomah County Division of Health Services. Both she and Ms. Johnson were members of the peer review committee.*

The commissioners responded by saying, "We're not paying you to just have nurses on the job," and, "we don't want people in high positions who aren't performing." The staff did not want that either, so the bargaining team said nurses would create a new evaluation system to go along with the pay scale, that the system would include specific steps and would guard against "just anyone" being promoted.

Over a period of one year, a committee of seven nurses developed three different evaluation tools. One, a nursing performance evaluation, is completed by the supervisor. Two, a self-evaluation, is completed by the nurse. Three, the peer review, is completed by peers. Peer review focuses on the nurse's relationships and leadership potential, not her practice in general. All three evaluations—supervisory, self, and peer—are done yearly. For newly hired nurses, they are also done after four and one-half months. In this article, we will discuss only one form of evaluation, peer review.

CATEGORIES TO MEASURE

The committee began by selecting 10 facets of interpersonal communication: cooperation, self-expression, originality and independence of thought, emotional maturity, initiative, capacity for advancement, sensitivity, knowledge and resourcefulness, reliability, and flexibility and adaptability. The nurses realized that communication skills play an important part in developing relationships and that, if these could be measured, persons could gain insight into their own style of relating and perhaps improve their own relationships.

The committee then wrote assessment factors for each of the 10 areas. Those for sensitivity serve as an example: allows others the opportunity to express feelings; suggests solutions in nondomineering and nonthreatening manner; is aware of own feelings and group feelings; listens to expression of feeling; and recognizes importance of nonverbal communication.

Percentages were assigned to those assessment factors for rating purposes. After many revisions the following scale evolved.

Score   Frequency of Performance
1—Less than 65% of the time
2—65 to 74% of the time
3—75 to 84% of the time
4—85 to 94% of the time
5—95 to 100% of the time.

All staff who are involved in the peer review are called the "peer group." This peer group includes all community health nurses in a supervisory area. Because we use the team approach, community health workers, licensed practical nurses, and secretaries who work with the nurses are included in the peer group, if these workers choose to do a review. In such cases, they also receive peer reviews. Because some nurses, such as coordinators, belong to no supervisory group, nursing administration requests at least 10 persons with whom they have worked closely to do a peer review.

REVIEW PROCESS

The supervisor sends out the forms, which peers complete anonymously and return in an envelope marked "personal." A secretary tallies the averages and the supervisor writes a summary of written comments and counsels the nurse on the results. The nurse keeps one copy and signs one, which goes into her personal file. This process takes about one month.

Nurses work together in many situations, so their observations of peers are by no means limited to a period of working at their desks before they start their day's visits. Nurses work with each other in well-child, immunization, hypertension, and family planning clinics. Nurses also co-lead various types of groups, such as behavior modification for preschoolers and creative parenting. In these settings, the nurses are able to evaluate the communication techniques their peers use with clients.

All nurses work together using the team concept in community health. Teams are small, three to six nurses per team. These teams share geographical areas of varying sizes, depending on number and economic status of the population.

The teams meet weekly to discuss plans for delivery of health services, hold case conferences, and divide the new referrals. The nurses write their own team plans using problems, objectives, and productivity indicators. The county's plans are used as a guideline, but the teams directly control how they will solve problems.

RESPONSES TO REVIEWS

Nurses have expressed both positive and negative feelings about peer review during the first year. Because the concept of peer review was brand new, there was great fear of the unknown. There were such comments as, "I hope this gives me input on promotion." "It's just a pecking system." "They'll just put me down." "I'm scared, but willing to try." "But they really don't know the real me." "I'd like to know if my peers see me differently than I do."

After everyone had been through peer review, nurses made such comments as, "It has given me input on promotion." "Can it be optional?" "I don't think I learned anything that I didn't already know about myself." "It lets you know your strong areas." "I think some people didn't take enough time in completing them, that is, didn't take them seriously enough." "I've seen my peers working on improving areas." "I think it's great." "It increased my self-confidence."

FOR NEGATIVE REVIEWS

At this time, there is no uniform procedure for a person to take if she receives a negative peer review. However, according to administration, reviews are seldom negative. If one examines closely the rating system, this can easily be explained.

The peer review and its rating system are designed to give positive feedback to the nurse. The percentage scale is set up so that all but rating number one shows that a person does the assessed factors at least 65 percent of the time. This is over half the time, so any of the scores cannot be considered negative.

Nevertheless, the lowest score of any review, whether it is 3.3 or 4.6, might be considered a negative by the person reviewed.

Various options are open to the nurse, but it is up to her to pursue them. One action would be to work with the supervisor at regular counseling sessions on ways to change behavior.

Another possibility would be to silently work on the desired areas for a time and then request another review from peers.

A third option, which may prove to be the most effective, is to take the results of the peer review to the area nurses for discussion. Although the resulting dialogue may seem frightening, some nurses have found such discussions helpful.

NURSE. *One area of my peer review that I would really like to work on is "needs to suggest solutions in nondomineering and nonthreatening manner." I did not realize that I came across in a domineering and threatening way, but obviously the group sees that in me. To help me accept this, can you give me some specific examples.*

PEER. *I remember when we were making out team nursing care plans. You made several suggestions that, I felt, we had to accept, or you would no longer cooperate. (Others gave more examples.)*

NURSE. *It is hard for me to believe; it was not my intention to come across that way. Can the group give me some suggestions on how to improve this area?*

PEER. *How about checking out your suggestions with the entire group before making them seem so mandatory, like taking a concensus?*
PEER. *How about saying, "What do you think of . . .?" rather than, "The only way to do it is . . ."*
NURSE. *These are all good suggestions, but sometimes I may forget them. I wouldn't mind being confronted at the time with something like, "Wait a minute, I feel threatened by what you are saying. Let's discuss that further."*

Each group is different, and there would have to be a high sense of trust in the group to do this. The Multnomah County staff have access to many mental health counselors and psychiatric nurses, who are skilled in group counseling and are good group facilitators. The nurse may want to invite one of these "outsiders" to come and lead the group so that all feelings and discussion can be handled in an appropriate way.

Another part of the entire evaluation packet is the nurse's self-evaluation. This includes the nurse's goals and objectives for each year. We hope that the staff nurse will include areas of her peer review in her goals for the year, admitting that she desired growth in areas of weakness her peers have identified.

Again, we emphasize that peer review is only one tool of three completed for each nurse yearly. All three are used as a basis for promotions.

Multnomah County has, at this writing, been doing peer reviews for one year. A new committee has been formed to review and revise the present evaluation system. Peer review must be kept up-to-date to meet our changing needs.

From *Nursing Outlook* 25:330-332, May 1977. Copyright © 1977. AJN Co.

A Statewide System of Record Audit

GRACE LOHMANN

Based on regional design and committees, this nursing care audit system resolved distance and peer review problems for small rural home care agencies.

Like other states, Iowa has seen a rapid development of home care programs in its rural areas. Usually, these services are provided by small agencies, most of which are official county health units employing one or two nurses. Consultation and inservice education are available to these agencies from the nursing section of the state department of health through six regional offices, staffed by 12 regional nurse supervisors, each of whom covers seven to nine counties.

The state health department is also responsible for certifying agencies which provide home health services for persons eligible under the Health Insurance Benefits Program (HIB). Since these agency services must be surveyed at regular intervals for compliance with HIB standards—for instance, those governing nursing and auxiliary services provided—it became evident that the agencies needed assistance in improving record keeping and in establishing a record review.

As a first step in conducting a statewide inservice program, the nursing section and the Blue Cross of Iowa, the fiscal intermediary for the HIB program, co-sponsored a series of workshops on documentation and recording throughout the state, reaching the staff of all certified home health agencies. The nurses attending the workshops expressed a desire to learn how to conduct nursing audits. As a result, another series of workshops was arranged and was again co-sponsored by the health department, the Blue Cross, and the state's assembly of home health agencies.

GRACE LOHMANN, R.N., B.S.N., *is a regional nurse supervisor with the Iowa State Department of Health, Des Moines.*

AUDIT METHOD SELECTED

The nursing audit developed by Maria Phaneuf was selected as the method to be used at the workshops, because of its relative simplicity.* It could also serve as a supervisory and staff tool and was appropriate to the agencies' needs and their staffing patterns. Phaneuf's audit form includes seven main areas to be judged and criteria for the subdivisions of each area. Each of these subdivisions receives a score which, when totaled, can point out strengths or weaknesses in the seven main areas.

The first of the auditing workshops was specifically planned for the regional nurse supervisors and was conducted by two consultants who were familiar with the Phaneuf system. Since this group of nurses would be responsible for teaching staff in their respective regions, it was considered essential that they develop expertise in conducting nursing audits. Additional workshops throughout the next year were given to staff from voluntary community nursing agencies and official county units. As part of the preparation for attendance, each agency staff agreed to study Phaneuf's book and to read articles from a prepared bibliography.

Implementing a statewide nursing record review system was the next step. Since this would be done at the regional level, two problems had to be considered: the size of the agencies, and the distances separating them from each other and from the regional supervisors' offices.

In 1972, when the workshops were held, public health nursing services were available in 80 of the 99 counties of the state. The number has increased; now 93 counties have such services. Seventy-six of the 83 official county agencies currently operating employ one to three nurses, while seven have four to five nurses. In addition, many of the voluntary and hospital-based home care agencies employ a small staff.

Peer review by one's co-worker was ruled out as one means of conducting audits, as it could scarcely be considered objective. On the other hand, using the regional supervisors for record audit was believed to be not only wasteful of the supervisors' time but also ineffective, in that those giving the patient care would not be involved in the review process.

Distance was another factor. Most of the rural agencies are 30 miles apart, although they are usually located in the county seats. Even though the regional supervisor is centrally located within a group of counties, some agency staff must travel distances ranging to 250 miles roundtrip to attend regional inservice or committee meetings. Mileage costs and the time involved, therefore, were important considerations.

---

*PHANEUF, M. C. *The Nursing Audit: Profile for Excellence.* New York, Appleton-Century-Crofts, 1972.

AUDIT BY COMMITTEE

During the last four years, however, a variety of methods have been used to conduct audits, and some patterns have evolved. The predominant one is the committee system. The following are some of the variations we devised.

• In one region, two committees, each with six or seven members, include all the nurses from three adjoining county agencies and several representatives from a visiting nurse association in that area. The committees meet with the regional supervisor at a central location for a day on alternate months. Each nurse brings one open and one closed record, which are exchanged. Then the nurses work in pairs to audit them. They discuss nursing care problems and share possible solutions.

• In two other regional areas, nurses from two agencies in adjoining counties alternate visits to each other's offices on a quarterly basis. They exchange records—usually several records per nurse—and conduct audits. This plan includes a small visiting nurse association, a hospital-based home health agency, and a certified homemaker health aide service. Both discharge and open records are audited.

The two supervisors in this area do not regularly meet with the committees, but review audit reports and discuss problem areas when they visit each agency. They also review current records periodically on their visits. One five-nurse agency in one of these regions audits its own records, with some assistance from the agency's professional advisory committee.

• In the northwest region, where each supervisor serves eight counties, committees are composed of nurses from four adjoining counties. When an agency employs more than one nurse, the nurses take turns attending meetings. One of the committees meets every three months with the regional supervisor and audits records from all of the eight counties. On those occasions, two open and two closed records are selected by each nurse for review.

• In another region, because of distance, nurses either send photocopies of records to the supervisors or the supervisors pick them up when they visit the agencies. These records are then distributed to staff at other agencies and are audited at the agency. Ten percent of the records in the total home care caseload can be followed using this system. Two visiting nurse agencies have joined the system.

• In another instance, two committees, each composed of half the nurses of the county agencies, take turns meeting with the supervisor every three months to audit all the records, both open and closed, for the region.

• In another plan started recently, a supervisor takes records from one agency to the next one she visits, at which time she and the nurses do the audits. This "round robin" plan is one more example of how to overcome the distance problem.

PROBLEMS AND SOLUTIONS

Although there were problems getting started, the committee system has worked well, and time and travel have been kept to a minimum. Most committees report that a six-member group has proved efficient. A larger committee, they believe, encourages "visiting" and often poses the problem of finding suitable work space. They also suggest changing the membership periodically, as it is difficult to remain objective year after year.

Other suggestions include not auditing alone in the agency's office, because interruptions and work demands usually take precedence. Setting a deadline for returning audit reports has proved to be an effective time-saver and motivator.

Plans for orienting new staff also must be made. Often this can be done during a committee meeting, or the supervisor who audits a record can review procedures with a new nurse. Some regions bring new nurses together for the orientation. Most new members require time to become adept and committee work may be slowed as a result, but all agree that the learning is worth the time.

Most committees have had problems interpreting audit items and reaching a uniform definition. Regional inservice meetings, at which everyone audits or re-audits the same record, have been useful in clarifying differences.

Finally, the fears expressed by some supervisors as well as staff that feelings would be hurt by audit scores and comments did not prove to be a problem as anticipated.

SOME RESULTS

When we started the audit system, documentation of the nursing process took the form of narrative accounts, which were often lengthy, time-consuming to read, and difficult to follow. These narratives became even more lengthy as efforts were made to correct deficiences and omissions that were found. The inadequacy of the forms was clear.

After a period of experimentation with new forms, a revised record system was adopted for statewide use by county agencies. The new forms make the organization of data easier and have improved the recording of the health history, assessment of patient's condition and family situation, problems identified, and plans for nursing interventions. Nursing actions and observations are recorded on a flow sheet. Only changes in the patient's condition, reactions, attitudes, or family situation and the results of teaching are described in the narrative recording. Some of the voluntary nursing agencies adopted our new forms or revised their own.

Changes in nursing care have occurred as recording has improved. Much more attention is given to obtaining a complete medical diagnosis and health history. Better ways for obtaining the renewal of physicians' orders were also developed. The identification of all medications taken by the patient, including self-administered medications, as well as the observation of possible reactions and interactions, were recognized as important nursing responsibilities and are now included in the record.

Assisting the family and patient to make plans for medical emergencies that might arise was seldom considered prior to the audit system, but the revised data base form includes this component. The actual plan decided upon, however, is recorded in the narrative notes.

Peer review has helped the nurses recognize both their strengths and weaknesses in providing care. The nurse who works alone particularly values the opportunity to discuss nursing care problems with associates. When the regional supervisors return audited records to an agency, they review them with the nurse responsible for the patient's care and focus on the findings. Weaknesses that continue to need attention include understanding the nurse's role in providing emotional support to the patient and family and helping the patient understand and adjust to his condition.

Many of the regional inservice programs are focused on learning needs identified by the audit process or are planned at the request of the nurses. For instance, in one region the older nurses asked for a program on fluid and electrolyte balance. Results of the learning were quickly evident in the improved recording of signs and symptoms of imbalance in the emphysematous or cardiac patient. Such evidence suggests improvement in the quality of care provided. Other sessions have been directed to a specific disease process and the nursing care required.

Another positive indicator is that audit scores have steadily improved, with the greatest increases occurring during the first six months of initiating the audit system. In one region, average scores improved from a low of 119 to 173 (out of a possible 200) over a three-year period. Most records now receive a high rating.

When statistical summaries for the region are compiled following committee sessions, these summaries are shared with all the participating agencies. Some supervisors develop graphs to compare the scores. As the nurses become more experienced as auditors, they become more proficient practitioners and more is expected of them.

One outgrowth of the record audit has been the development of standardized nursing care plans. A committee of supervisors identified 24 common disease entities or conditions for which such care plans seemed appropriate. Each supervisor chose two or three conditions from the list and, with staff from the agencies in their area, developed a care plan for patients in each category. A standardized format recommended by the committee was followed. Eventually this material was compiled and distributed to the agencies for use as a reference.

CONCLUSIONS

Those of us involved in the record audit system believe it has functioned well. It has provided a means of peer review for many small agencies and has upgraded the quality of nursing care given. We believe our system could be used in other areas of the country with rural areas and many small home care agencies.

REFERENCES

1. MAYERS, M. G. *A Systematic Approach to the Nursing Care Plan.* New York, Appleton-Century-Crofts, 1972.
2. SCHELL, P. L., AND CAMPBELL, A. T. POMR—not just another way to chart. *Nurs. Outlook* 20:510-514, Aug. 1972.
3. PHANEUF, M. C. Analysis of a nursing audit. *Nurs. Outlook* 16:57-60, Jan. 1968.
4. RUBIN, C. F., AND OTHERS. Nursing audit—nurses evaluating nursing. *Am. J. Nurs.* 72:916-921, May 1972.
5. DAUBERT, E. A System To Evaluate Home Health Care Services. *Nurs. Outlook* 25:168-171, Mar. 1977.

From *Nursing Outlook* 24:107-109, Feb. 1976. Copyright © 1976. AJN Co.

Health Record Students in a Home Health Agency

BROOKE BRANON • JUDITH WEILERSTEIN

The benefits to both agency and school were many when these specialized students had field experience in a visiting nurse association.

Home care agencies, like all other groups involved in the delivery of health care, are becoming more and more conscious in this day of accountability of the importance of the documentation of care, development of adequate statistics, and the necessity of carrying out quality assurance studies. Many hours of valuable professional time are spent in attempts at designing forms and statistical reports. This is usually done on an as-needed basis, with little thought to using the skills of those knowledgeable in system technique, forms design, and quality assurance methodology. However, an opportunity to collaborate with specialists in record management presented itself to our agency.

Representatives of our visiting nurse association were asked to share information about their patient care recording system in a seminar on innovative record systems sponsored by the Western Pennsylvania Medical Record Association several years ago. Through their attendance at this seminar, they met a faculty member of the Department of Health Records Administration in the School of Health Related Professions, University of Pittsburgh.

MISS BRANON *(B.S.N., Hartwick College, Oneonta, N.Y.; M.S., Graduate School of Public Health, University of Pittsburgh) is associate director in the Visiting Nurse Association of Allegheny County, Pittsburgh.* MISS WEILERSTEIN *M.P.H., School of Public Health, University of Pittsburgh, Pa.) is a registered record administrator and was assistant professor in the department of Health Records Administration, School of Health Professions, University of Pittsburgh, when this article was written. She is presently director of the medical record program at Northeastern University, Boston, Mass.*

The university program was designed to prepare health (medical) record practitioners, who would be knowledgeable in the documentation of care wherever it was given and committed to professional participation in all types of health agency record activity. The curriculum includes courses in community aspects of health care, systems analysis, health statistics, information retrieval, health law, and quality assurance. Its graduates become, after completion of a national qualifying examination, Registered Record Administrators (RRAs). Most of the graduates of this type of program are employed in hospital record departments; others in a variety of health-related activities requiring expertise in record management.

ADVANTAGES TO AGENCIES

The benefits of an alliance between the university and the VNA was apparent to both agencies. The visiting nurse association could benefit from skilled record consultation (which it could not afford to purchase), and the university would have an excellent opportunity to provide its students with a clinical experience that would introduce them to an important component of health care and help them gain insight into the problems of illness. It would also give them the opportunity to use their professional skills in an underdeveloped area of health record activity.

A contract for field experience between the nursing agency and the university was agreed upon. A faculty member would serve on the agency's professional advisory committee and offer some professional consultation, and the agency's education coordinator would participate in the university's academic program. Each student experience would be for a minimum of three days and include home visits, observation of the record system and clerical functions of the agency, and orientation to the specific activity either selected by or assigned to the student as his course project. The students were expected to complete their projects independently after the field experience, only visiting the agency when necessary. Satisfactory completion of the projects would be predicated on faculty and agency approval.

PROBLEMS IDENTIFIED

Agency personnel easily identified an abundance of possibilities for student projects. Many suggested areas in which they thought help with records was needed and posed specific questions for which they were seeking answers. The difficulty was to sort through the problems and establish priorities. The areas identified were so many that projects for every member of the class could have been established, if this had been feasible from the point of view of either the school or the agency. It was the role of the instructor to identify specific projects that students could handle within the broader concerns of the agency, priority of need, skills of the students, value of the learning experience, and time constraints.

In the first year, four students were assigned to such topics as the refinement of diagnostic categories, revision of forms, data collection on stroke groups, and utilization review. This was so successful that during the second year, seven students were assigned to four more projects: record audit, development of a statistical system for a homemaker program, development of a central intake and referral system, and research into the need and potential role of a health record administrator in the VNA program.

STUDENTS' PROJECTS

Now after two more groups of students have completed their experience, we can see that although the projects varied, systems studies were the major focus. Some examples of the student projects follow.

The VNA had a number of regional offices around the city. Staff at each office took information on new referrals or prospective cases; however, this information remained in each office. There was no master index of patients within the agency, thus making it difficult to gather information about types of patients or staffing needs or patterns. Two students undertook a study of the feasibility of a central intake register.

They charted the flow of the existing system and studied the volume and distribution of new calls. They also investigated existing technology for rapid information exchange, the cost of such, as well as the personnel and forms required. Their study led to the development of a logical system for the flow of information within the VNA.

All intake calls are now centralized and handled by one nurse and one full- and one half-time clerks. Information is transmitted to each regional office by a telecopier, which sends a facsimile of the copy of the intake record. The cost we have found is less than messenger service and is far more flexible than messengers.

The students also analyzed cases not accepted or visited and found that it was difficult to group information according to established checklist categories. Comments on these records had to be interpreted, leading to marked variability among the data collectors. After discussion with the professional staff, the categories were explicitly defined and this information given to those collecting the data.

A second major area of student activity has centered on the design and revision of record and data gathering forms. While the VNA has an excellent and unique basic patient record format, its total system includes a melange of special projects for which documentation was poor. Students have designed and tested forms for collecting information for such diverse areas as stroke patients and the number and type of guest observers visiting the agency. Their study of employment application procedures has resulted in a revised application form and a new form to document career mobility within the agency. In addition, they examined turnover rate in the homemaker-home health aide program. As a result, the administrative staff of the agency restructured the basic recruitment activities for these workers. Recently, forms and statistical tables to document the agency's Affirmative Action program were designed.

Students have also been involved in quality assurance activities, which have included the design of utilization reports, abstracts, and procedures and methods for selecting statistically valid samples for audit. One student elected to use the agency for a much longer—90-hour—independent project that is another requirement of the school. She wished to test use of the recent DHEW publication, "Patient Classification System for Long-Term Care," as an audit tool. She plans to see if this method of classifying functional status is useful as an audit mechanism. The student, working under the guidance of the assistant director of the agency, has tested the classification system on many patients' records to see whether the record, as constituted, supplies the needed information.

She found that many specific items asked for on the audit form were not readily available on the record; that is, mobility level was only determined on 8 percent of the charts, although walking was recorded on 88 percent. The greatest deficiency was in relation to the description of patients' behavior patterns and orientation to time and place, or risk factor measurements; only blood pressure was charted often enough to be counted.

A recommendation was made that an initial patient assessment form be developed that includes only those items that are considered essential to the treatment plan. Then an audit can be made of the functional status of the patient in relation to the information obtained on the assessment. It was also suggested that the nurses develop criteria for patient teaching and emotional support of patients and include these in the audit.

Students are also involved in administrative studies. Two students took as their project a study of medical record services in the VNA. Based on their findings they recommended use of a part-time RRA consultant to work on record policy, evaluation of the overall information system, and review of other record activities. They also recommended hiring an ART—(Accredited Record Technician—graduate of a two-year community college program) who would be responsible for carrying out day-to-day record activity, supervision of clerical personnel, participation in studies, and so forth. These recommendations have been adopted in part—an RRA has been employed full time by the VNA.

The school will continue to supply professional consultation. Indeed, it hopes to find a way to expand its relationship with the VNA and undertake a more detailed evaluation of their entire information system, both patient and management.

CONCLUSIONS

The agency and school believe that this is a useful program. The needs of both groups have been met with relatively little effort. The agency has been able to secure assistance in looking at some of its information handling problems, and the school has been able to provide its students with an opportunity to participate in a type of health record activity not usually open to them.

We believe that there has been relatively little contact between home health agencies and the health record profession. We feel that the health record professional, with a dual background in health care and information handling, has much to offer agencies involved in health care delivery. Better understanding and collaboration between both groups have the potential of improving care for patients through a more efficient use of our resources.

From *Nursing Research* 25:252-255, July-Aug. 1976. Copyright © 1976. AJN Co.

Community Health Nurses' Preferences for Systems of Protection

PAT M. KEITH • MARY CASTLES

This study examined community staff nurses' and nursing students' preferences for escort protection in areas in which they would refuse to go alone and investigated the nurses' comfort in performing tasks in the presence of a protector.

Recent studies have documented nurses' fear of the environment in which they work(1-5). Various means of coping with fear have been proposed. In addition to education about the community through seminars and field experience, efforts to change attitudes, and counsel about dress and appearance, escort service has been suggested as a technique for managing fear.

Other occupations which are organized in a dyadic one-to-one client-professional relationship are being altered to attain security. Social workers, police, teachers, and more recently psychiatrists have established role relationships which provide protectors. One possible ramification of adopting systems of protection is the decrease in privacy between client and practitioner while work tasks are being completed. Although Hughes implied that workers in most occupations prefer not to be observed by clients and peers(6), little information is available on the

PAT M. KEITH *(Ph.D., Saint Louis University, St. Louis, Missouri) is associate professor of sociology, Iowa State University, Ames.* MARY M. CASTLES *(Washington University School of Nursing, St. Louis, Missouri; Ph.D., Saint Louis University, St. Louis, Missouri) is associate professor of nursing, College of Nursing, Wayne State University, Detroit, Michigan.*

extent to which professionals endorse the use of protectors or their perceptions of working in the altered setting.

This study—which considered community nurses' preferences for various systems of protection (in this case, types of escorts) to be employed in areas in which they would refuse to go alone—investigated the influence of type of agency, student-staff status, role performance, and evasion on preferences. Whether nurses would be comfortable performing nursing tasks in the presence of a "protector" also was studied.

Method. Nursing students (N = 53) and staff nurses (N = 106) in an official (governmental) community health agency and a nonofficial (nongovernmental) community health agency responded to a questionnaire administered in groups. Eighty-one nurses were employed in the official agency, and 78 respondents worked in the nongovernmental organization. Nursing roles in the two agencies differ. In the official agency, the main task of the community health nurse is teaching; a primary function is education and counseling regarding health care. The nurse has an official mandate to prevent illness in the community. Home visits are likely to be initiated by the nurse as a part of her regulatory responsibility. This is in contrast to the nurse in the nonofficial agency who goes into the home at the request of the patient or his doctor, and whose work entails skills and techniques related to physical care, assessing patient needs, monitoring and coordinating care, and making referrals.

Individuals were asked to respond to each of several systems of protection in terms of whether they would be: 1) willing to go into a community with protection where they would refuse to go alone; 2) comfortable carrying out their nursing duties in the presence of various types of protectors.

The four types of protection which respondents were to accept or reject, derived from responses to open-ended questions by another sample of nurses in a pilot study, were presented as follows: 1) a driver takes you to your destination, waits until you are in the building, and picks you up when you come out of the patient's home; 2) a nurse stays with you during the home visit; 3) a member of the community meets you when you enter the community, remains during the visit, and stays with you until you leave the community: 4) a hired bodyguard, who is not a member of the community, remains with you until you leave the community.

To assess role performance and evasion, nurses were asked whether they would refuse to make a home visit to provide care to a patient because of the characteristics of the community in which he was a resident. From responses to this question, two major categories of role behavior were delineated: 1) role evasion, manifested by individuals who would refuse to accept a patient for care because of the characteristics of the community in which he lives, and 2) role performance, expressed by nurses who would accept a patient for care regardless of the characteristics of his environment.

Findings. *Status.* An initial exploratory consideration—that nursing students would prefer types of protection that would enable them to maintain a detached position, a low level of peer and supervisory visibility, and, thus, maintain the "idealistic" one-to-one nurse-patient relationship described by Davis *et al.*(7)—was supported to the extent that students tended to reject systems of protection which entail visibility of performance and endorsed a system which enables them to function without peer visibility.

Table 1. Endorsement of Systems of Protection and Perception of Comfort in Work of Nursing Students (N = 53) and Staff Nurses (N = 106) in Number and Percent

SYSTEM OF PROTECTION	ENDORSEMENT OF SYSTEM OF PROTECTION					PERCEPTION OF COMFORT IN WORK				
	STUDENTS		STAFF		χ^2	STUDENTS		STAFF		χ^2
	N	(%)	N	(%)		N	(%)	NM	(%)	
Driver	31	(58)	28	(26)	13.44**	—	—	—	—	—
Nurse present	24	(45)	67	(63)	4.41*	32	(60)	83	(78)	5.86*
Community member	25	(48)	61	(58)	1.39	26	(49)	65	(61)	1.85
Bodyguard	10	(19)	51	(48)	9.53**	5	(10)	45	(42)	16.25**

*p = .05
**p = .001

Table 1 reveals significant differences in student-staff preferences for systems of protection on three of the four types. Employment of a driver to the client's home received the greatest student endorsement with preference for use of a bodyguard being the least attractive alternative. Nurses, however, preferred to be accompanied by a colleague and were least likely to want a driver who waits until their work with the client is completed. Subjects differed significantly on perceptions of their comfort in carrying out nursing functions in the home accompanied by another nurse or a bodyguard (Table 1). Students indicated they would be less comfortable than staff working in the presence of either a bodyguard or a nurse. Although greater proportions of staff believed they would experience no discomfort with a member of the community present, the staff-student difference was not significant.

Table 2. Endorsement of Systems of Protection and Perception of Comfort in Work Situation by Role Behavior in Number and Percent

System of Protection	Endorsement of System of Protection				Perception of Comfort in Work Situation				
	Evasion		Performance		χ^2	Evasion		Performance		χ^2
	N	(%)	N	(%)		N	(%)	N	(%)	
Driver	26	(41)	34	(36)	0.38	—	—	—	—	—
Nurse present	38	(60)	51	(54)	0.45	52	(82)	62	(65)	4.55*
Community member	36	(56)	50	(53)	0.11	37	(58)	52	(55)	0.07
Bodyguard	27	(42)	30	(31)	1.68	22	(35)	24	(26)	1.33

*$p = .05$

Thus, on five of the seven items, there was support for the assumption that nursing students would be more likely than staff to reject systems which entail visibility of performance and endorse a system which would enable them to function without peer visibility.

Role Behavior: Performance and Evasion. In response to questions regarding role behavior, 64 respondents, described as role evaders, would make care for a patient contingent on his community of residence. The remaining 95 respondents who would not use geographical location as a basis for refusing patient care were designated as performers.

Table 2 shows that evasion and performance did not directly affect preferences for systems of protection, and only one item dealing with perceptions of comfort in performing nursing functions, i.e., presence of a nurse, was associated with role behavior. Although only one of the seven items was significant, there was a trend for greater proportions of evaders to endorse alternative systems and perceive themselves as being at ease in the presence of protectors.

When evasion and performance were introduced as controls, relationships between status (student—staff), preferences, and perceptions of comfort remained unchanged except student evaders were more similar to staff members than student peers in their willingness to endorse the presence of a nurse and perception of comfort in carrying out nursing duties in her presence (Table 3).

Further analysis which examined within-status differences, e.g., student-student, while controlling for role behavior (evasion, performance), indicated evasion and performance differentiated the preferences of nursing students on two systems of protection, i.e., acceptance of a driver and being accompanied by a nurse. Student evaders were significantly more likely (78 percent) to approve a driver than were their counterparts who

Table 3. Endorsement of Systems of Protection and Perception of Comfort in Work Situation by Status and Role Behavior in Number and Percent

System of Protection	Endorsement of System of Protection						Perception of Comfort in Work Situation					
	Evasion			Performance			Evasion			Performance		
	Student	Staff	χ^2	Student	Staff	χ^2	Student	Staff	χ^2	Student	Staff	χ^2
	N (%)	N (%)		N (%)	N (%)		N (%)	N (%)		N (%)	N (%)	
Driver	15 (78)	10 (23)	14.77***	18 (47)	16 (28)	7.6**	— —	— —	—	— —	— —	—
Nurse present	13 (67)	26 (57)	0.48	13 (33)	39 (69)	9.9**	15 (83)	36 (80)	0.07	18 (47)	44 (77)	8.07**
Community member	10 (56)	26 (56)	0.00	17 (43)	34 (60)	2.08	11 (56)	26 (59)	0.06	17 (46)	35 (62)	2.30
Bodyguard	5 (22)	22 (53)	4.55*	6 (17)	23 (40)	4.80*	2 (11)	20 (47)	6.86**	4 (9)	21 (38)	8.9**

*$p = .05$
**$p = .01$
***$p = .001$

are performers (47 percent, $X^2 = 4.48$, $p < .05$). Endorsement of a driver by evading students accounted for some of the magnitude of the student-staff difference on this dimension. Both the continued presence of a nurse (67 percent, evaders; 33 percent, performers) and perceived comfort in this situation (83 percent, evaders; 47 percent, performers) were endorsed significantly more often by student evaders ($X^2 = 5.23$, $p < .05$; $X^2 = 6.25$, $p < .02$). On these dimensions, the evading nursing student resembled her staff counterparts more than student peers who opted for role performance. There was considerable agreement among student evaders and performers on all items related to employment of members of the community and bodyguards.

When staff preferences were examined further, controlling for evasion and performance, role behavior was not associated with any of the seven categories of staff preferences for systems of protection or perceptions of the work situation. Thus, the general trend for evaders to endorse protectors and have positive perceptions of working with them, based on the simple crosstabulation, can be explained in part by differences within the student sample.

Table 4. Endorsement of Systems of Protection and Perception of Comfort in Work Situation by Type of Agency in Number and Percent

System of Protection	Endorsement of System of Protection			Perception of Comfort in Work Situation		
	Official	Nonofficial	χ^2	Official	Nonofficial	χ^2
	N (%)	N (%)		N (%)	N (%)	
Driver	32 (39)	29 (37)	.08	—	—	—
Nurse present	43 (53)	48 (61)	.94	53 (65)	62 (79)	3.51
Community member	42 (52)	51 (66)	2.53	36 (44)	55 (70)	8.94*
Bodyguard	30 (37)	27 (34)	.00	18 (22)	34 (44)	6.50*

*$p = .01$

Type of Agency. Responses to alternative systems of protection were also considered in terms of the two types of agencies—official (governmental) and nonofficial (nongovernmental)—in which the nurses and nursing students were employed.

Crosstabulations revealed no significant association between type of agency and preferences for systems of protection (Table 4). However, type of agency was significantly related to perception of the work situation on two of the three items. Nurses in the nonofficial agency were more likely to believe they would be comfortable working with a member of the community or a bodyguard, and there was also a trend ($X^2 = 3.51, p < .10$) for them to indicate they would be at ease with a nurse present. This suggests that differences in work activities noted earlier may influence anticipated adjustments to protectors.

Controlling for type of agency, only four items showed significant differences between student-staff preferences. Type of agency did not help explain student-staff differences noted earlier in preferences for a driver, being accompanied by a nurse, or perceptions of working in the presence of a nurse. However, the data suggested that greater staff preferences for and comfort with a bodyguard occurred in the official agency where there were significant student-staff differences on both dimensions, whereas nursing students and staff in the nonofficial agency had more comparable preferences (Table 5).

Preferences within status groups (e.g., student-student) were considered by type of agency. Type of agency did not discriminate between student preferences on any of the 14 items and only one of the staff responses. Staff in nonofficial agencies were significantly more likely to indicate they would feel at ease in the presence of a member of the community. Crosstabulations of student-staff preferences, controlling for both role behavior and type of agency, showed that the positive perceptions about working with bodyguards and community members held by persons in nonofficial agencies were independent of student-staff status or role behavior.

Table 5. Endorsement of Systems of Protection and Perception of Comfort in Work Situation by Status and Type of Agency in Number and Percent

System of Protection	Endorsement of System of Protection						Perception of Comfort in Work Situation					
	Official			Nonofficial			Official			Nonofficial		
	Student	Staff	X^2	Student	Staff	X^2	Student	Staff	X^2	Student	Staff	X^2
	N (%)	N (%)		N (%)	N (%)		N (%)	N (%)		N (%)	N (%)	
Driver	23 (54)	8 (22)	7.46*	10 (73)	18 (29)	7.54*	— —	— —		— —	— —	
Nurse present	20 (47)	23 (59)	.94	4 (31)	42 (66)	3.38	24 (58)	29 (72)	1.66	10 (64)	51 (82)	.96
Community member	19 (46)	23 (59)	1.18	7 (54)	44 (68)	.72	18 (43)	18 (46)	.04	10 (64)	44 (71)	.25
Bodyguard	8 (19)	22 (56)	10.43**	3 (18)	24 (38)	1.60	2 (5)	16 (40)	12.85**	4 (21)	26 (44)	2.28

*$p = .01$
**$p = .001$

146

Discussion. In contrast to the role of the nurse in an institutional setting, supervisory and peer visibility are at a minimum for the community health nurse. For the nurse who anticipates and is attracted to community health nursing because of the greater degree of autonomy and discretion which accompany low peer visibility, a system of protection may be perceived as a hindrance(7).

The suggestion, that nursing students would prefer systems which enhance autonomy, decrease peer visibility, and preserve the one-to-one nurse-patient relationship, tended to receive support. Students, regardless of type of agency or role performance, preferred a driver who would not be present during their work with the client.

Projected role behavior in the form of performance and evasion was more influential for students than for staff. Although anticipated evasion by students resulted in their greater endorsement of a driver, the most crucial distinction between evading and performing students seemed to be their preferences and attitudes toward another nurse. Students fearful enough to opt for evasions were willing to forego the one-to-one relationship and accept the presence of a nurse in exchange for greater security. Being fearful of certain aspects of a community, as expressed in evasion, however, did not increase the willingness of nursing students to endorse a bodyguard. Use of a bodyguard may run counter to idealism atttributed to students.

That persons in the official agency believed they would be more uncomfortable working in situations that involve protection than their counterparts in the nonofficial agency may be explained in part by the difference in the role they perform. Nurses in the nonofficial agency who are requested to come into the home and who perform a standard, technical skill in physical care may be less reluctant to have their performance observed than their counterparts in the official agency who perform what may be idiosyncratic teaching and regulatory functions. These tasks are of a more particularistic nature, the procedures more ambiguous, and the outcome less certain.

As noted earlier, Hughes suggested that workers in most occupations prefer not to be observed by clients and peers(6). In an area of indeterminate technology (such as that of the teaching function of the community health nurse in an official agency) evaluations and assessments of laymen, e.g., protectors, become more salient. Perhaps individuals in occupations with a less well-developed technology tend to value highly the luxury of privacy in making and correcting mistakes and are less at ease in situations in which there is an increase in peer or lay visibility. However, visibility may be viewed as an opportunity. Low visibility may restrict learning the content of a job or the possibility of having one's "good" performances viewed favorably(8). With reference to differences in student-staff preferences for protection, perhaps staff with more confidence in their expertise perceive high visibility as a way to get favorable feedback to superiors. On the other hand, nursing students who have less experience and fewer skills may be more reluctant to perform in the presence of superiors or peers who are in a position to judge their behavior.

The data provide some direction for adoption of alternatives. Although there were significant differences in the extent to which staff and students shared perceptions about working in the presence of a colleague, within both groups this system of protection received the most support as providing a positive setting for performing nursing functions. However, systems involving members of the community also appeared to be viable options. While systems incorporating a member of the community did not receive the largest percentage endorsements by nurses or nursing students on either dimensions of preference or comfort, there was least discrepancy between responses of the two groups on this alternative. Employment of a member of the community would be less costly than a nurse, would free a nurse for other activity, and would, possibly, at the same time, avoid the stereotype of confrontation which a bodyguard might evoke. For some individuals, systems of protection may seem impractical and not cost-effective. Yet, costs relative to increased delivery of service need to be assessed. Increased quantity and improved quality of service may outweigh the additional expenditures.

We have, however, treated only individuals' preferences for modes of adaptation to the work environment. Utilization of systems of protection would require altered philosophic and task commitments and a change in resource allocation, alluded to above, on the part of health organizations. Data from respondents indicated that frequently organization policy is to ignore or not acknowledge that fear is an aspect of working relationships. Nevertheless, data show that fear(4) and danger(5) are facets of the role of the public heath nurse in metropolitan areas.

While a manifest function of the systems of protection is to lessen fears about performing in a threatening environment, at the same time they may also increase visibility and subsequently decrease inactivity or partial role performance due to fear. Concomitantly, the uncertainty and anxiety experienced by individuals who perceive themselves vulnerable to a hostile environment, but who are willing to utilize a system of protection, would be somewhat reduced, and greater efforts could be concentrated on the performance of skills.

REFERENCES

1. CASTLES, M. M., AND KEITH, P. M. Correlates of environmental fear in the role of the public health nurse. *Nurs. Res.* 20:245-249. May-June 1971.
2. KEITH, P.M., AND CASTLES, M. M. Impact of environmental fear on public health nurses. *HSMHA Rep* 88:201-204. Mar. 1973.
3. _____. Agencies in cities in crises: A descriptive study of selective characteristics. *Am. J. Public Health* 63:46-51, Jan. 1973.
4. FITZPATRICK, LOUISE. Safety and the community nursing experience. *Nurs. Outlook* 19:527-531, Aug. 1971.
5. MULLIGAN, JOAN. Agencies in cities in crises: A descriptive study of selective characteristics. *Am. J. Public Health* 63:46-51, Jan. 1973.
6. HUGHES, E. C. *Men and Their Work.* Glencoe, Ill., Free Press, 1958. pp. 88-101.
7. DAVIS, FRED, AND OTHERS. Problems and issues in collegiate nursing education. In *The Nursing Profession: Five Sociological Essays,* ed. by Fred Davis. New York, John Wiley and Sons, 1966, pp. 138-175.
8. THOMPSON, J. D. *Organizations in Action.* New York, McGraw-Hill Book Co., 1967.

Section IV Home Care: An Alternative to Institutionalization

The articles in this section describe a variety of schemes for providing home care for patients who would otherwise require extended hospitalization or institutionalization. Often, home care is administered by a hospital; at other times, the coordination of a multitude of community service agencies is necessary to ensure the adequacy and effectiveness of the home care program. The community health nurse frequently is the professional who coordinates and manages such care efforts.

From the *American Journal of Nursing* 75:1811, Oct. 1975. Copyright © 1975. AJN Co.

Hospital-Based Home Care

MILDRED HORN

Bringing the hospital to the patient offers therapeutic
resources without expensive in-hospital residence.

Home is where the heart is—the heart of providing health-oriented, humane care for patients who do not require hospitalization.

Home is where a patient enjoys the warmth, dignity, and privacy inherently lacking in an institutional residence. At home a patient is with family and friends, aided in his daily living and spiritually reinforced by them. More important, he convalesces more rapidly and retains his independence longer and more positively in familiar surroundings.

Home care costs can be a small fraction of institutional fees. The hospital and nursing home fee of $50 to $300 per day can be avoided. And what about skilled nursing and other therapies? These can be provided by hospital-based staff, going into homes as needed. The total resources of the hospital can be called upon for consultation and assistance. Complete patient records are readily available.

With clearly apparent advantages, it is difficult to justify the slow growth of hospital-based home care. It is not keeping pace with the mushrooming expansion of health care facilities.

Hospital-based home care must be sold to the people capable of giving it life and growth: physicians, hospital trustees, administrators, insurance companies, government, and, not least of all, patients. Physicians find the hospital locale more convenient with better control of patients; hospital administrators can hardly be expected to promote business away from hospitals; intermediaries find home care procedures hard to audit; and the general public is hardly aware that home health programs exist.

MILDRED HORN, R.N., *is director of Home Health Services at Lake Forest Hospital, Ill.*

Current hospital-based home care agencies exist in a variety of modes from modest inhospital-quartered teams of a few nurses to independently headquartered administrations keyed to serving multihospital geographical areas. Holding together such a multidisciplined web is a highly sophisticated communications system.

At Lake Forest Hospital, the inhospital-administered home care program accepts patients by direct inhospital referral as well as posthospitalization referrals. It is centrally administered under the control of the board of directors of the hospital.

The coordinated planning, evaluation, and follow-up procedures provide hospital services to patients at home: nursing care, physical therapy, respiratory therapy, speech therapy, nutritional guidance, hospital equipment, Homemaker-Home Health Aide, laboratory services, medical supplies, social service, family therapy, legal counsel, Home Meals, Telecare, volunteer services, community referrals, pharmacy (patient drug profiles), and consultation from such hospital departments as business and administration and other available services.

A professional advisory committee, representing every medical department, each therapeutic service, and consumers, suggests policy.

The home care staff is employed by the hospital and thus benefits from continuous hospital inservice education conferences, seminars, and workshops. They also serve on such hospital committees as new products, procedures, medical audit, and utilization review.

The home care nursing staff also rotate annually through the different hospital care units—coronary care, for example—to keep up with the fast moving technology of therapy.

Herein lies the great potential of hospital-based home care—the best therapeutic skills as needed but without expensive inhospital residence.

Hospital home care programs have a high degree of surveillance, care, and control through intimate communication links between patients, nurses, physicians, therapists, and other hospital specialists. This availability of counsel is a product of the personal contact between people who operate under one roof.

From *Nursing Outlook* 24:625-630, Oct. 1976. Copyright © 1976. AJN Co.

Comprehensive Home Care
for Earlier Hospital Discharge

ELAINE McCARTHY

*A coordinated multi-agency and multi-service pro-
gram led to centralized care, supervision, billing, and
cost and resulted in savings to both patient and
insurers.*

The young woman had been in the hospital seven weeks. Originally admitted to give birth to her first-born—a healthy girl—she developed a
series of complications and was becoming depressed and apathetic. Her
husband had lost his job and was at home caring for the baby. This was
the first referral made to the Coordinated Home Care Program—a multi-
agency, multi-service program initiated by our VNA—by a head nurse
who said, "Here, see what you can do with this one. We're not getting anywhere with her."

The patient's physician gave his approval to plan for care at home and
estimated that three more weeks of hospitalization could be saved by
such a plan. The visiting nurse-coordinator assessed the patient's needs
and financial resources and interviewed the husband, the hospital nurse,
physical therapist, social worker, and three physicians who cared for the
patient.

Then patient and visiting nurse mapped out a home care plan that included nursing care, supervision of medications, home health aide service, physical therapy, laboratory work, and transportation to the doctor's
office. Social service follow-up was planned for assistance with financial
and employment problems.

ELAINE McCARTHY, R.N., B.S.N., *is director of the home care program
described here and based at the Visiting Nurse Association of Milwaukee,
Wisc.*

The transition from dependent patient to mother at home was a painful one. The relatives expected more of the woman than she was able to give; the baby was turned over to her for night feedings. The visiting nurse continued to work closely with the mother and in five weeks of comprehensive service our first case turned into our first success. Follow-up hospitalization for further testing was cancelled by the physician; office visits were sufficient. Recovery seemed complete—in fact, surpassed expectations.

START OF THE PROGRAM

The concept of coordinated home care is not new; many visiting nurse associations (VNAs) provide supportive home care services, but mainly for post-hospital and chronic stages of illness and for a limited number of services. The VNA of Milwaukee was interested in developing a competent, comprehensive, multi-service program that would reduce the cost of health care, shorten hospitalization, and hasten recovery—all through one centralized service. This would mean one telephone call by a patient or physician to order a variety of services. It would also mean centralized billing, better follow-up of the services, one bill to patient and insurance providers each month, and fairer cost of vendor services.

The Milwaukee VNA was chosen by the United Community Services to plan and implement such a multiple service program, and a state grant was secured to survey existing services throughout the country. The Rochester, New York, Organized Home Care Program was particularly helpful in giving suggestions and encouragement. The VNA then conducted a survey of the kinds, quality, and cost of services available in our city. This alone was an eye-opener; there were more health services available than anyone expected. Agency ego had led us to believe that we were providing most of the services people needed, which was not necessarily true. Actively ill patients required a broader spectrum of services than we offered.

We also found that there were no standards for cost or quality of services offered by private vendors. For example, checking with three laboratories, we found that a complete blood count (CBC) ranged in price from $3.50 to $12.50; patient equipment was not always sent out in the cleanest or best condition, and so on. Fortunately, however, Milwaukee had every health service necessary to carry out an independent and complete home care program. The VNA drew up a proposal for a program in 1969, and it was approved by the local Blue Cross, medical society, regional medical program, hospital council, and the comprehensive health planning agency. Funding to get the program started was provided by the

Faye McBeath Foundation, United Community Service, and the VNA auxiliary. An administrative team—consisting of a medical director, nurse director, and social worker—was appointed in mid-1971 to implement the program.

FINANCING AND CONTRACTS

Located at the VNA, the administrative team's first concern was to secure a financial base, which was done through a contract with Blue Cross that covered 100 percent of the program. The contract also defined services to be provided in the program. The VNA's attorney was employed to draw up contracts for vendors of service and for hospitals wishing to participate in CHCP. Several hospitals knew of the VNA's proposal; three had their own home care programs on a smaller basis. At first, four hospitals requested to participate in the program; now nine hospitals are involved in the program.

Financial advisors assisted us in establishing fees based on predicted costs, as well as a centralized billing system that was separate from the regular VNA caseload system. An administrative fee of $5.00 per day, regardless of whether the patient was seen or not, was established. This fee covers the cost of the administrative team, the coordinator's assessment, weekly reports which are sent to the physician, hospital, and insurance provider. It also covers the centralized billing, other clerical expenditures involved in coordinating care, keeping controls on vendors, and maintaining proper utilization of services. This fee was based on prorating all the services given. As our volume of patients went up, the administrative fee went down. The administrative fee was based on the Social Security cost study and the National League for Nursing cost analysis. In addition, the vendors chosen to provide services for CHCP patients were eager and cooperative in meeting the standards VNA requested. The competition gave us the benefit of price and quality control.

STAFF RESPONSIBILITIES

Besides the administrative team, the staff consists of four VNA nurse coordinators and two secretaries. Other VNA services are given by the staff of 75 RNs, three physical therapists, two social workers, and a nutritionist. In addition, 25 home health aides are available through the agency, and two proprietary agencies supply aides on call. In order to have uniformity of standards, a select number of home health aides from proprietary agencies have received inservice at VNA. They work with patients under a visiting nurse's supervision.

The medical director's role is administrative and he serves the entire agency. He has a private practice and spends an average of four hours weekly at the VNA. He interprets CHCP functions to the medical staffs at the hospitals, is spokesman for CHCP, and reviews patients' progress records at the weekly multi-disciplinary utilization conference. In the process of these reviews, he observes the patient's response to treatment and use of services. If there is any problem with medical direction from a patient's physician, he will phone and speak to the physician.

The nursing director supervises the nurse coordinators' activities; screens the referrals for the type of nursing input and coordination of services needed; is the VNA spokesman for the program; interprets CHCP to nursing staffs and community groups; participates in the weekly review of patients' progress; and supervises the use of nursing services.

The social worker assists the coordinators in patient assessments when necessary and provides service directly to patients at home or indirectly by offering guidance to the staff nurse upon request. Since the CHCP is a short-term care program, the social worker primarily refers patients to community services that will provide long-term care. She provides short-term counseling on such things as financial aid and long-term planning. To our surprise, this worker has had a significant number of requests for marriage counseling for those over 65 years.

If a hospital social worker has been involved with a patient in any depth, the CHCP social worker will deal directly with that worker in order to have a complete history and smooth carry-over of the services. She also assists the visiting nurses with discharge planning, if necessary, and reviews the patient's weekly progress along with the medical and nursing directors.

Coordinators are visiting nurses who have had at least two years experience on staff. They are particularly skilled in assessing and interviewing and are "quietly aggressive." Each coordinator has at least two hospitals that she visits on a regular weekly schedule. At these times, she screens potential patients and interviews hospital staff. The job of nurse coordinator has been deliberately left as unstructured as possible to give the coordinator freedom to function where she sees the need. She does not do staff nursing in the field. If there is a lull in referrals, she will call one of the three VNA offices and offer help. The coordinators are invaluable; they are the public relations people and VNA representatives in the hospitals and community.

Two clerks assist in coordinating services. Initially, an RN had been considered essential for taking all referrals and ordering equipment and supplies. We found, however, that the secretaries easily learned to elicit medical details needed for basic referral information, which they then relay to a nursing supervisor. Another advantage of using secretaries instead of nurses is that they are less inhibited when it comes to bargaining with vendors for a deal in cases where the patient has no health insurance coverage.

In addition to taking referrals, the clerical staff do insurance checks so the coordinator will know what services are or are not covered at the time she is discussing home care with a patient. The secretaries also order all services for patients prior to admission and as long as the patients are in the program, and handle all billing procedures and any complaints about equipment and supplies. All patients receive a letter upon admission to the program and are given a number to phone if they have any problems. Either the secretary will handle the problem or refer the patient to the appropriate supervisor.

CRITERIA FOR ADMISSION

Although exceptions are sometimes made with approval by the administrative team, all patients considered for the CHC program must meet the following criteria. Each patient must (1) be in a hospital participating in the CHCP; (2) have his physician's approval to participate in CHCP; (3) be considered an early hospital discharge; (4) need an acute or intermediate level of care, or require care because of an exacerbation of a chronic illness; (5) have consented (as well as family member or caretaker) to the CHCP plan; (6) be able to be adequately cared for at home—that is, the home environment must be conducive to recovery; and (7) not require 24-hour skilled care. Referrals of patients in nonparticipating hospitals are sent to the regular VNA program; however, that program does not have the benefit of a patient assessment before hospital discharge or coordinated services that are billed centrally.

The usual means of securing referrals is prompted by the nurse coordinator who will approach the patient's physician and suggest what CHCP has to offer patients who appear to be good home care candidates. Once familiar with the program, physicians often make their own referrals. It also helps if their patients have praised the home care services. In approving the referral, the physician agrees to provide on-going medical direction but is not expected to make house calls. The doctor will also certify the estimated number of hospital days saved. Usually, this time is not fewer than seven days or more than 60 days.

If a patient is rejected, the coordinator will put a written notice to this effect on the patient's chart, including the fact that the patient's status was assessed, the reasons he was rejected for the program, and the nurse's recommendations for an alternate plan of care. These recommendations may include continued hospitalization, referral to a nursing home or rehabilitation center, or to a social or some specialized community agency.

The hospital nurses and physicians did not take kindly to having their referrals rejected, but these rejections have had a positive effect. They prevented the VNA from being used as a dumping ground when no other discharge planning had been done for the patient, or having a caretaker overwhelmed with care that he or she was incapable of giving. They also prevent a patient from being placed in an unsafe or poor home situation and offer better alternatives. In turn, this helps hospital personnel to become more aware of other community resources. In addition, the written rejections have been used by utilization review committees to document that the patient needs longer hospitalization. They have also helped to increase the integrity of the coordinator's professional judgments, particularly in those instances when patients were sent home in spite of their rejection for CHCP, and they had to be returned to the hospital.

SERVICES OFFERED

Patients are provided with a variety of services, which are recommended by the patient's physician and the nurse coordinator. These include professional nursing care, as well as home health aide service. The latter is provided only as long as personal care is needed and includes meal preparation and light housekeeping. Supportive services include physical therapy, social service, and occupational, speech, and inhalation therapy. Also available are laboratory testing and EKG, portable x-ray, hospital equipment and supplies, prescription drugs (covered by Blue Cross and some private insurances), ambulance or other transportation; and mobile meals (covered by Blue Cross only).

Payment for these services varies with the insurance provider. Each patient is made aware of the provisions of his individual policy benefits, whether it is private insurance, Medicare, or Medicaid. Occasionally insurance does not cover the full cost of the services needed. Some patients choose to remain in the hospital, if too many expenses would accumulate on home care. For those who prefer home care but are not covered by insurance, a fee based on a sliding scale is set with the patient. The coordinator also uses all available community resources to help meet patient needs in cases of financial hardship, particularly for those under 65-years of age.

MECHANICS OF COORDINATION

Each hospital participating in the program has a liaison person with whom the VNA coordinator relates. It might be a social worker, nurse, discharge planner, or the head nurse on each hospital unit. Ideally, the liaison person reviews the Kardex at regularly scheduled times with the head nurse on each unit. Potential early discharge patients are brought to the coordinator's attention when she makes her scheduled hospital visits; however, anybody can intiate the referral. Some have come from sympathetic cleaning women, policemen, and hospital visitors who have seen our brochures or posters. The coordinator reviews all the cases brought to her attention. Once the physician's approval is obtained, the coordinator visits the patient to discuss home care. At the same time, an insurance check is made to find out what services will be paid for at home. Blue Cross in Milwaukee will allow the patient 100 percent coverage for the hospital days he has left on his policy. If he is rehospitalized, the number of days in the CHC program will not be deducted.

If the patient agrees, an in-depth assessment then follows. All pertinent information in the patient's chart in summarized, as well as the patient's care and progress. Information is obtained from the nurse, physical therapist, inhalation therapist, social worker, dietician, or anyone else concerned with the patient. If possible, the patient will be observed in physical therapy or diabetic class, for instance, to assess his level of knowledge and to ascertain what reinforcement will be necessary at home. When the total needs are known, the coordinator will discuss a home care plan with the patient and caretaker.

Sometimes heavy equipment cannot be used in the home, or the family may not want it. If the caretaker has any unresolved misgivings about providing care, these concerns have to be dealt with realistically or there may be reason to delay the patient's discharge. Most patients are eager to go home and readily volunteer even the mailman as a caretaker! Occasionally, the coordinator will make a home visit to assess certain provisions or the safety of the home. In selected cases where there are complicated nursing procedures, the visiting nurse assigned to the patient will go to the hospital to observe the care. Once the home care plan is established, transportation is arranged to the home and the patient is seen the following day by the visiting nurse.

STATISTICS AND RESULTS

Based on our three years of experience, the patients' average length of stay in the program is 30 days. Home visits range from daily to once weekly, as the patient's condition stabilizes, and average one and one-half hours by the RN. During the past year, usually 55 patients were admitted each month, with a daily caseload of 40 patients. CHCP patients comprise 8 percent of the total VNA caseload and, in three years, 1,500 patients have been admitted to the CHCP. During 1975, the average cost per day was $18.00, compared to a conservative estimate of $175 in the hospital.

The diagnoses of patients vary, but the highest number are cancer (40 percent of total), followed by cardiovascular, CVAs, fractures, and other medical-surgical diagnoses. The high cancer rate can be attributed to the multiple cancer clinics in the area; many oncologists make referrals. The majority of these patients receive daily or weekly radiation or chemotherapy, and laboratory work is done in their home. Transportation to outpatient departments or doctors' offices is provided when necessary.

The age of patients ranges from newborn to 100 plus; however, 52 percent are over 65 years. One centenarian, whose age is unknown, recalls carrying buckets of water for General Lee's soldiers during the Civil War! The majority of patients discharged from the program are transferred to the regular VNA program. This means the patient's condition has stabilized, coordination of multiple services is no longer necessary, or the patient and family are better able to cope with the illness.

The program has benefited many—the hospital, the consumer, community, and VNA. In the hospital, it has improved communications between departments, reduced costs of the hospital handling its own home care program, improved continuity of care and the quality of discharge planning, and established mutual trust between hospital nurse and community health nurse.

From the consumer's view, the program has provided more than lip service to continuity of care; reduced anxiety and gaps in health care; enabled patients to leave the hospital early and convalesce more rapidly at home by providing intense services during the initial phase of home care; offered a direct route to other community resources; provided better quality of service at reduced prices; prevented hospital readmission or nursing home placement; and provided safe and supportive care on a one to one basis.

The community has also benefited because cooperative efforts of all available community health services are more potent than individual efforts. The program helped reduce the cost of health care and improved the standard of services available. In fact, it stimulated exceptional personal response from vendors. At the same time, the VNA gained, too. The program helped the agency to expand the skills of its staff and quality of nursing care it offered. It increased the staff, services, and patient caseload. In addition, the program broadened the age range of patients served and created greater community awareness and use of VNA services.

PROBLEMS AND LIMITATIONS

Because of the foundation laid so wisely and patiently by the board of directors and the executive director of the VNA, relatively few problems have arisen in a program as complex as CHCP. There are some limitations, however. For instance, I.V. therapy is not given at home and the demand for physical therapy has not been met because of a dearth of therapists in community health. Restricted funding has also limited the most needed services—homemaker-home health aide and transportation. Then, too, some patients with minimal home care insurance benefits have chosen to remain in the hospital rather than pay for a cab to the outpatient department, or because they cannot find or afford a housekeeper to prepare meals.

The problems we encountered during the past three years have been minimal but recurrent. Experience has taught us to assess more carefully and to recognize that we cannot be all things to all people. Some of these problems are (1) the family or caretaker misrepresented the amount of responsibility they were willing to take; (2) demand for service beyond what was assessed as necessary; (3) abusive attitude when the patient was not allowed to remain on CHCP until all his insurance benefits were used; (4) family or home situation not conducive to recovery; (5) unreasonable demands of a few physicians or their inaccessibility for further medical orders and supervision; (6) a higher rate of hospital readmissions in terminally ill patients; (7) retroactive denial of insurance payments of initially approved patients or those who appeared to be eligible for certain benefits; and (8) nonacceptance of the administrative fee and the health related services by some insurance providers.

CHANGING GOALS

The goals for CHCP have changed as we broaden our services and consider the needs expressed by the community and the users of the program. Use of PSRO in the hospitals will undoubtedly motivate hospital staff to accelerate referrals and refine discharge planning. Hospital care, too, will be geared to the acutely ill patient, and home care will become more sophisticated. As we review our present program, we believe patients could be admitted to the program without being hospitalized for intermediate care or diagnostic work. To do this, however, we will have to improve our present methods of identifying levels of care. We believe a community health nurse can also be called upon by a physician to do a patient assessement at home to determine the patient's needs and level of care, recognizing at the same time that home care is not always the best answer for all patients.

The rapidly increasing number of patients will present many new problems. For instance, how can the caretakers—whether family member, nurse, or home health aide—of the terminally ill be given more support?

How can we, or should we, prevent rehospitalization of dying patients, many of whom are sent back to the hospital only hours before death?

Another goal is to convince insurance companies to expand funding to those patients who are not acutely ill, but still too incapacitated to function self-sufficiently. Many of these patients could be maintained at home, but, without home care coverage, must be sent to costly nursing homes or hospitals for care.

Our last goal is to promote the concept of a coordinated health care plan and to contribute any information to other home health agencies interested in organizing a program of their own. We know our services have been appreciated, from evaluations we have requested from patients and participating physicians. Word of mouth has helped to expand use of our services more than any other means. To paraphrase one doctor's evaluation, "My patient received all anyone could expect and it was intelligently given. I plan to use it [CHCP] as often as possible." This accurately summarizes the majority of responses received.

It seems paradoxical that not so long ago people had to be convinced of the value of hospital care. Now we are struggling to convince them of the value of care at home. We are optimistic, however, in expecting a whole new era in home care and family involvement in that care.

From *Nursing Outlook* 23:570-573, Sept. 1975. Copyright © 1975. AJN Co.

Triage: Coordinated Home Care for the Elderly

JOAN L. QUINN

An institution may be the simplest solution for the care of the older person, but it is not necessarily the best. An alternative is care in the home, which is discussed here.

It's often easier to put someone into a nursing home than to arrange for the services necessary to keep him at home. The literature is filled with accounts of older people consigned to institutions who could, with supportive care, have remained in their familiar home environment. Among other considerations, the institutional route may go against the person's wishes, be more costly in the long run, and fail to meet the real needs of the individual. But the assumption has often been that once the older person is provided with the multiplicity of services available in an institution, he is well cared for.

In recent years, however, there has been some reversal of such thinking. There is growing awareness that institutional care is only one—and not necessarily the best—way to sustain the well-being of the elderly person. In line with this realization, the State of Connecticut about two years ago authorized a study to determine whether alternatives to institutionalization for the older citizen were available in that state.

The study revealed that the comprehensive services necessary to maintain such persons in their homes were not readily accessible. Furthermore, the ease with which an older individual could be permanently institutionalized contrasted sharply with the difficult negotiation through the complex, fragmented, and uncoordinated system necessary

MS. QUINN *(B.S.N., M.S.N., University of Connecticut, Storrs) is project director of Triage, described in this article.*

to maintain the person at home. As a result of these findings, the then newly legislated Council on Human Services for the state was assigned the task of sponsoring a pilot project to coordinate a system of care for elderly residents in their homes.

PILOT PROJECT

Under the aegis of this council, a three-year project was initiated in a seven-town region in central Connecticut.* The area includes both urban and rural districts of mixed ethnic composition and with a population of some 20,000 residents over 65 years of age. Project offices were established in Plainville, a town that is central to the other six towns in the region.

Thus Triage was born. Its name derives from a French verb meaning "to pick, to choose, to sort," and in essence that is what the Triage personnel do. The functions of Triage include full assessment of needs, nursing diagnosis, referral, and follow-up of older residents to assist in coordinated delivery of the full spectrum of care.

Another function has been out-reach case-finding but this has been minimal, for the referrals to Triage without much publicity have come in astounding numbers. It presently is receiving approximately 100 referrals per month.

SERVING THE ELDERLY

The Triage program is scheduled to run for three years, after which it will be evaluated and recommendations will be made. Currently it is in its first year of operation.

Often the first remark of an elderly client to the Triage representatives who visit him is something like, "I don't know how I am going to make it through this month." Depending on the individual, this same message is delivered with more or less eloquence, with more or less passion, but, nonetheless, felt and spoken.

For many, food costs alone are almost prohibitive. And when rent, utilities, and other so-called privileges such as a telephone are considered, many people are sorely pressed to find the resources to maintain themselves with any sort of dignity or peace of mind.

Since nutrition almost inevitably suffers when inflation mounts, and since many Triage clients lack the necessary health and stamina to do many ordinary household chores, the coordination of home-delivered meals has been a crucial part of the Triage contribution.

---

*Berlin, Bristol, Burlington, New Britain, Plainville, Plymouth, and Southington.

But the problem does not end with nutrition and inflation. It goes on into the realm of physical health, environmental needs, poverty of socialization, transportation.

Often this has meant providing a homemaker several times a week to do light housecleaning, wash clothes, and cook. One 81-year-old woman, living in housing for the elderly, has a homemaker who comes in at noon each day to prepare her lunch, make her bed, and dust the apartment. This service not only allows the woman to maintain her own home, but also gives her someone to talk to, someone she has come to depend on and trust as well.

Other Triage clients have received the services of home health aides, visiting nurses, and persons prepared to do household chores. Without Triage, it is safe to say that many of these people would not have received such services and perhaps would have been institutionalized by this time.

In the area of transportation, Triage has negotiated agreements with local public transportation companies and has provided the impetus for the granting applications for two new specially equipped vans to provide service to senior citizens.

Several weeks ago, for instance, one woman was faced with having to cancel a doctor's appointment because her daughter who usually drives her to the doctor was suddenly unable to do so. She called her caseworker at Triage to see if anything could be done on this short notice. Because of a prior agreement between Triage and a cab company, a taxi provided her with the necessary round-trip transportation, thus enabling her to keep her appointment.

THE ORGANIZATION

What is Triage and how does it function from day to day? The project director is a nurse clinician with a master's degree in nursing with a particular emphasis on gerontological nursing. In addition, there are five teams, each with a nurse clinician and a social service caseworker. There is also a community coordinator, whose functions include meeting with providers in the region to assist in development of new services and to draw up contracts for all services given to the Triage client.

There are also a fiscal and an assistant fiscal officer, responsible for grants management and the internal fiscal operation, and a secretary and a medical transcriptionist. All of these people are directly responsible to the project director. The staff salaries are paid by grant funds, primarily from the Title III, Older American-Act grants.

Five physician advisors, available to the Triage nurse-clinicians for consultation if medical problems arise, include a gerontologist, two internists, a physician whose specialty is chronic disease and rehabilitation, and a psychiatrist.

FINDING CLIENTS

Of course, the primary requirement for any such project is clients. How do elderly people find their way to Triage? Or, the other way around, how does Triage find those who need its help?

Most of those we serve come by direct referrals from community agencies and institutions. To date, there have been 27 different sources, including visiting nurse agencies, homemaker services, R.S.V.P. program, senior centers, state welfare department, clergy, social service department of institutions, and physicians. In addition, many elderly make the initial contact themselves.

There are also a large number of family referrals—not surprising when one considers that the average age of the clients we are serving is 77.5 years. Children of these older people are often approaching retirement themselves, and the responsibility of their parents' problems is more than they can handle.

PRIMARY OBJECTIVES

In outlining Triage, the planners enumerated six primary objectives.
- Provide a single-entry mechanism by which the elderly can have their physical, social, psychological, and life-support needs evaluated;
- Develop, through demonstrated need, necessary preventive and supportive services;
- Integrate the efforts of service providers to give coordinated care;
- Create financial support as needed for the full spectrum of services;
- Demonstrate the value of preventive and supportive services;
- Demonstrate the cost-effectiveness of coordinated care.

First, it seemed essential to have a mechanism that could funnel all the physical, social-psychological, and life-support needs through a single channel and, in turn, supply the services through this mechanism. A single entry system was developed, by means of which the needs of an elderly person could be evaluated by a routine procedure, as follows.

After a referral has been made to Triage, a geriatric nurse-clinician visits the client in his or her home to assess the individual's specific needs and decide what care plan is appropriate to meet them.

She uses a special assessment form that records the person's complete health and social history and includes an evaluation of housing, transportation, finances, and other social needs. A scale indicating activites of daily living, a mental status quotient, and other socio-demographic data are included.

Next, the nurse clinician performs a modified physical examination of the client which includes, but is not limited to, hearing and vision measurement, cardiopulmonary and musculoskeletal evaluation, and urinalysis. Any symptomatology mentioned by the client during the health history is further evaluated during the physical assessment. After this interview and assessment, all of the information obtained by the nurse clinician is organized and charted using Weed's problem-oriented approach.

A TEAM AFFAIR

Working as a team, the nurse clinician and the social worker then decide on the necessary services. If it is determined that the elderly person should not be institutionalized, the two health workers decide which preventive and supportive services the person needs to remain in a safe environment at home. Such services might include homemaker assistance, transportation, visiting nurse services, visits to a physician for further evaluation of medical problems, help with household chores, meals on wheels, friendly visits, telephone reassurance, laboratory studies, and/or weekly rides for isolated elderly persons living in single-family dwellings. Any or all of these services may be prescribed by Triage and delivered by providers of such service in the seven-town area served by Triage.

Institutionalization is sometimes prescribed as an appropriate placement for some elderly. The Triage team then works with family members to ensure that a placement is made that is acceptable to them and their elderly relative.

ARRANGING FOR SERVICES

The services prescribed are provided by existing service providers in the seven-town region. For example, if a client needs the services of a home health aide, contact is made with the visiting nurse agency that provides service in his town. The nurse clinician discusses the plan of care with the visiting nurse. If the client is eligible for food stamps, the Triage caseworker will help him fill out the application and see that he has transportation to obtain the food stamps.

The client might also be lonely and isolated. The caseworker would then refer him to the R.S.V.P. program for friendly visiting and would try to see that the friendly visitor and client had mutual interests. As a result of the continuing client-nurse-caseworker contact, the services can be changed as indicated.

A health service report is returned to Triage monthly by the service provider who is assisting the Triage client. This report tells the staff how the elderly client is responding to the service and also mentions significant information about his health or social status.

Necessary life-support services are also integrated to avoid duplication of use. For instance, when the nurse clinicians realized that many of the Triage clients would be on special diets, likely service providers to be approached were the two general hospitals in the region who had dietitians on their staffs. These institutions also produced large numbers of meals. Triage then drew on the state service funds to help the providers develop the meals-on-wheels service.

The nurse clinician assesses, prescribes, and directs the care given to elderly recipients. It is then up to the caseworker to arrange for delivery of the services and to keep in touch with the client at home or in an institution to ensure that the services provided are adequate and appropriate. Even when no services are necessary, the caseworker maintains client contacts.

COORDINATED CARE

One of the objectives of Triage is to integrate the efforts of service providers to give coordinated care. This integration is being accomplished through both the single-entry assessment mechanism, as described, and by the planning and activities of the Triage board of directors on which all health providers in the region are represented. Included are five visiting nurse agencies, two homemaker agencies, three acute care hospitals, and one chronic disease and rehabilitation hospital.

Seven elderly consumers, one from each town in the central Connecticut region, are also members of this board, as is the Triage director. Discussion at monthly advisory board meetings addresses regional needs of the elderly, services presently being provided, and those new services which need to be developed in order to keep a person at home.

In addition to seeing that the elderly person receives care, Triage helps pay for the necessary care if the client is unable to. Triage will subsidize the costs with special funds it has been granted for that purpose. No client is denied help because of his inability to pay.

In all cases, Triage tries to avoid spending for unnecessary services and care. It is hoped that this will allow third-party funds (Medicare, Medicaid, and private insurance) to cover the more basic and correct needs at the appropriate level. Medicare and Medicaid are now available to clients, but there are many constraints, such as amount of service delivered as well as determination of eligibility for services.

An example might be a 75-year-old woman whose fractured right arm is immobilized. After two weeks of home health aide service, it was determined by the Medicare fiscal intermediary that she no longer needed skilled nursing care, so the service was terminated. Her arm was still in a cast, however, and she still had difficulty dressing, bathing, and preparing her meals. But the assistance was not there.

Triage intervened in this case by prescribing that the services of the home health aide be continued for two hours each day for the next four weeks until her cast was removed. If the extension of the service had not been provided, the client might well have ended up in a rest home at a much greater cost. In this instance, Triage was able to help because it receives grant funds direct from the Administration on Aging through its Older American's Act and state monies for services from the Council on Human Services.

A prepaid contract with the state welfare department is also in operation.

The services prescribed will most likely be needed on a long-term basis or for an indefinite period. The nurse clinician/caseworker teams expect that the optimum outcome for clients through Triage intervention is to maintain them at their present, relatively stable status. As the client grows older, the normal aging process will undoubtedly impose more disability, and his need for services in the home may very well increase. Certainly, over time, an older individual will not need fewer services.

LIFE WITH DIGNITY

So many older people come to feel that as they grow old they have lost their value, and once they feel that way, the inevitable result is depression and a bitter death. If ever there is a goal in working with the elderly, it must be to allow each to feel the worth of life, the goodness of his humanity, the love of himself and other people, and ultimately to die a death with dignity.

Who can help to make this possible for those who are pained and bitter and despairing? Other people—people who love and care. A case in point is Nicholas, a 76-year-old, Russian-born man, recently widowed, who told the nurse-clinician during the initial assessment that he was lonely and depressed.

He delighted in receiving a telephone call that was a wrong number because he could always try to strike up a conversation. Daily contact by phone and a twice-monthly visit by the caseworker resulted in the following response made to the caseworker, who had become his friend.

Not long ago I was angry and depressed and feeling sorry for myself, and I only wanted to die. But now I want to live, at least to see another spring and summer. And then, then if God wants to take me, I will let him, and I will be happy and at peace.

A nurse clinician who functions as both administrator of the project and clinician in the field is a relatively new concept in the state and the local region. Nurse clinicians manage and direct the assessment teams and provide the patient's primary care. There is often unique entry into the heath care system, as the nurse clinicians are often in the position of uncovering pathology that the elderly client might ascribe to "old age."

The success thus far of the project is being looked at closely by the state. The use of Triage as a model by which health care can be delivered throughout the state for all age groups is the eventual goal.

FURTHER PLANS

We also hope, through Triage, to demonstrate by documentation the value of basic preventive and supportive services and to demonstrate the cost-effectiveness of coordinated care.

These objectives will necessarily have to be looked at over time. As the project has just ended its first year of operation, it would be premature to state results.

However, the value of the services received by the Triage elderly in the form of supportive services, as well as preventive services, has been voiced eloquently. For Mr. C, 80 years old, who lives with and cares for his 75-year-old hemiplegic wife, Triage assessment and referral for services have made life "much easier." The care of his wife is shared by Mr. C and a home health aide. Home-delivered meals have made him feel better and given him more time to devote to his wife's care. The stress of his supporter role has been mitigated considerably.

Most of all, he and his wife are in their own home together, and care is being prescribed and delivered according to their individual needs. Although in this case it is still too early to evaluate the financial cost-effectiveness of their coordinated care, the emotional cost-effectiveness is evident in the improvement of the quality of their life.

From the *American Journal of Nursing* 76:762-764, May 1976. Copyright © 1976. AJN Co.

Outreach to Welfare Hotels, the Homebound, the Frail

PHILIP W. BRICKNER • ANNE G. BOLGER
SISTER MARY T. BOYLE • SISTER TERESITA DUQUE
PATRICIA HOLLAND • JAMES F. JANESKI
ARTHUR KAUFMAN • PATRICIA M. MADDEN

An urban medical center's community programs for three population groups vary, but nurses are primary care providers and decision makers in all three programs.

Current hospital practice is designed with the expectation that sick people will go the source of health care. Many people, however, cannot or will not use this established health care system. Among these medically unreached groups are derelict, homeless men; homebound sick people; and the aged who have borderline physical capacity(1-6).

Through the Department of Community Medicine at St. Vincent's Hospital of New York, we have brought professional services to these medically unreached groups for the past six years. Physicians, nurses, and social workers from the hospital work in close association with the Visiting Nurse Service of New York and community groups and individuals. Success has depended, to a major degree, on the planning ability and independent role of nurses as health workers(7).

The three outreach programs in which we have demonstrated nursing in coequal roles with medicine are (a) the welfare hotel programs for derelicts, (b) the Chelsea-Village program for the homebound aged, and (c) the nurses' clinic for the aged persons who are severely restricted but not literally homebound.

WELFARE HOTEL PROGRAMS

Urban derelict men are a group apart from the rest of the poor(4).

Generally too indifferent, frightened, or angry to seek help when ill, they often receive no care. In 1969, nurses from the Visiting Nurse Service of New York and physicians from St. Vincent's Hospital began a clinic at a hotel that housed about 1,200 men. It was located in a middle-class residential area of Greenwich Village on the lower west side of the borough of Manhattan.

The New York City Department of Social Services used the hotel to house destitute, homeless men. There was a rapid turnover of residents, but the men could be divided into three general categories: about 200 were aged men, about 450 were middle-aged alcoholics, and more than 500 of them were young men addicted to heroin.

Many of the 200 aged men had lived at the hotel for decades. Most lived precariously on social security payments or welfare. Some had menial jobs.

The middle-aged alcoholics were unemployed and living on welfare. They differed from the classical skid row man only in that they were able to stand erect.

The young heroin addicts at the hotel had recently been released from prison and had no legitimately acquired funds other than from welfare. The younger, more aggressive men used the others as prey.

The clinic for these men, in three small connecting rooms, was operated four or five afternoons a week. No fees were accepted and no registration procedure took place, although visits were recorded.

Men who wanted medical care simply appeared at the clinic or the nurses found them during their tours of the hotel rooms. The nurse or physician obtained a history, if possible, performed a physical examination, and gave advice or treatment.

Most patients were under the care of both a physician and a nurse. The physicians, with their greater experience in physical examination and

Six of the authors are staff members of St. Vincent's Hospital and Medical Center, New York, N.Y., or of its school of nursing. PHILIP W. BRICKNER, M.D., is director, Department of Community Medicine; and SISTER TERESITA DUQUE, R.N., is nurse-coordinator, Ambulatory Service Programs. JAMES F. JANESKI, M.S.W., M.P.A., is assistant director, Department of Community Medicine. SISTER MARY T. BOYLE, R.N.; PATRICIA HOLLAND, R.N., B.S.N.; and PATRICIA M. MADDEN, R.N., are instructors in the School of Nursing. ANNE G. BOLGER, R.N., M.A., is a supervisor at the Lower West Side Center of the Visiting Nurse Service of New York. ARTHUR KAUFMAN, M.D., assistant professor of family and community medicine, University of New Mexico School of Medicine, was formerly a resident physician at St. Vincent's.

The authors acknowledge with gratitude the support of their work by the New York City Department of Health and the United Hospital Fund of New York.

diagnosis, were often consulted by the nurses for more complex medical problems. The nurses excelled in case finding and long-term treatment, often against great patient resistance.

A nurse found A.B., a 65-year-old man, and induced him to come for treatment. A massive leg ulcer, due to venous stasis, trauma, and neglect, involved the entire anterior and lateral surface of his left leg below the knee.

After the initial evaluation, the nurses took over full care of this patient. He often refused soaks and antibiotics but the nurses persisted and, after 10 months, new epithelium covered the lesion and the ulcer was considered cured.

During the 18 months the clinic ran, 309 patients were seen a total of 1.117 times. At length, community opposition to the presence of the men rose to such a height that the New York City Department of Social Services moved them to flop houses on the Bowery or to other parts of the city(1). We continue to conduct similar clinics in other smaller welfare hotels in our part of Manhattan.

THE CHELSEA-VILLAGE PROGRAM

In January 1973, we started the Chelsea-Village program, designed to reach aged, abandoned, homebound patients in Chelsea and Greenwich Village, the area St. Vincent's Hospital serves.

Failed physical capacity forces many urban old people to suffer a hazardous existence alone in single rooms and welfare hotels. Poverty is a common additional disadvantage. These people are often too disabled, frightened, or confused to seek help. We estimate that some 3,000 to 5,000 such people live in our part of Manhattan, unable to leave their rooms because of illness or fear. These are "hidden" people who have outlived or been abandoned by family and friends.

Members of local churches, settlement houses, block associations, tenants' councils, and police precincts serve as case finders of these hidden patients.

Physicians, nurses, and social workers from St. Vincent's Hospital go to the patients, as needed. The professional staff, who work on hospital time and with the hospital's support, volunteer for this service. The hospital gives comprehensive care when necessary, but our ultimate aim is to keep our patients out of institutions, in their own community, adequately housed, and healthy. Our program operates without cost to the patient.

These people's complex difficulties are often a mixture of medical, psychiatric, social, financial, and housing problems. A physician's ordinary house call, even if it were readily available, would not fulfill their needs. The combined skills of our staff and the assistance of community people are necessary.

In the first three years, 347 people (232 women, 115 men) received 2,110 visits. The oldest was aged 105, the youngest 24, and the average age was 79.

The nurse is a key figure in the success of the Chelsea-Village program. This job is currently filled by a registered nurse who is also a Sister of Charity. She evaluates referrals and regularly makes screening visits to determine patients' needs for services from other program staff.

She also performs a full variety of nursing activities in patients' homes. In addition, she functions as a nurse practitioner for a selected group of our patients who do not need or who refuse additional medical or social service.

The nurse is generally known and trusted in our community and is in a position to solve many difficult human issues. These often relate to patients' fears regarding the power of a large institution, such as the hospital, to dehumanize and manipulate individuals.

M.C. is an 83-year-old woman who lives in a senior citizen's hotel, out of contact with relatives. She had been highly suspicious of people who attempted to help her, and was not being treated for her chronic congestive heart failure.

The hotel manager requested attention from the Chelsea-Village program. After the initial evaluation, the patient would accept visits only from the nurse. As a consequence, for 24 months she has carried health care responsibility for this patient, including interval physical examination and control of medications. She regularly discusses the case with a physician. The patient is thriving.

NURSES' CLINIC

The third program is for the many aged people who, while not literally homebound, are severely restricted in their activities. These people commonly lack regular access to medical care, but are able to seek assistance to a degree.

Through contact with a large local senior citizen's center, the Fulton Senior Center or Hudson Guild, we established a nurses' clinic in October 1973. This unit meets weekly at the center and is staffed by two to five senior nursing students from the St. Vincent's Hospital School of Nursing, with direct supervision by two instructors.

The purpose of the clinic is to provide members of the Fulton Center with free, easily accessible, basic preventive health care and health instruction. During the first two years of the clinic, the nurses saw 612 patients in 1,860 total visits. At each visit, patients see the same staff team. Appointment lists are made when possible, as reminders of need for follow-up and to distribute the case load. The students stated in their initial report:

We sat down and talked and listened and tried to find solutions (to the patients' health problems) which were within their means. We did not act as physicians. We checked diets, exercise limitations, and, most important, medications. Medications were an area which we thought required much teaching.

For medical consultation, physicians from St. Vincent's attend the nurses' clinic on request. The nursing students believe that this work enables them to develop a sense of independence in nursing judgment, acquire new methods of communication, and broaden their understanding of disease entities and their effects on the total person.

In each of these three ongoing community health care programs, the nurse's role and the nurse-physician relationship differ. In each, however, nurses have achieved an independent status.

In the welfare hotel programs, the nurse and physician function as coequal partners in patient care. The patients are often difficult to deal with and cooperate poorly. Mutual support by the professional staff is particularly important.

The Chelsea-Village program also deals with complex cases, but the nurse has ample opportunity to act as an independent health professional in planning, decision making, and evaluation. The nurse has a case load of about 10 patients for whom she is the primary provider.

The nurses' clinic is an opportunity for nursing students, under proper supervision, to experience the wider field of practice which will be open to them as nurses. A physician enters into patient care only on specific request. The students have the opportunity to gain the self-confidence that is essential to the nurse practitioner.

In all three programs, nurses function as independent health workers and have coequal responsibility with physicians in planning, decision making, and evaluation.

REFERENCES

1. BRICKNER, P. W., AND OTHERS. A clinic for male derelicts; a welfare hotel project. *Ann.Int.Med.* 77:565-569, Oct. 1972.
2. BRICKNER, P. W., AND KAUFMAN, A. Case finding of heart disease in

homeless men. *Bull. NY Acad. Med* 49:475-484, June 1973.
3. BRICKNER, P. W. Finding the unreached patient. (editorial) *JAMA* 225:1645, Sept. 24, 1973.
4. BLUMBERG, L. U., AND OTHERS. The skid row man and the skid row status community. *Q.J. Stud. Alcohol,* 32:909-941, Dec. 1971.
5. BRICKNER, P. W., AND OTHERS. The homebound aged: medically unreached group *Ann.Int.Med.* 82:1-6, Jan. 1975.
6. SOMERS, A. R., AND BRYANT, N. H. Home care: much needed, much neglected. (editorial) *Ann.Int.Med.* 82:111-112, Jan. 1975.
7. BRICKNER, P. W. Expanded roles for nurses. In *Changing Role of the Hospital and Implications for Nursing Education.* Papers presented at the annual meeting of the Council of Diploma Programs held at Kansas City, Mo., May 1-3, 1974, (NLN Pub. No. 16-1551) New York, National League for Nursing, 1974, pp. 1-4.

From the *American Journal of Nursing* 76:1789-1791, Nov. 1976. Copyright © 1976. AJN Co.

Respiratory Care at Home

BOBBY L. MALKUS

All a patient with emphysema asked was to go home to die. His eventful rehabilitation shows how a visiting nurse association's respiratory home care program gives disabled people fuller lives.

Two young women in Hanover General Hospital, Pennsylvania, would need artificial ventilation at least part of each day the rest of their lives. Who could provide it? Seeking an alternative to prolonged hospitalization, the director of the respiratory care service, Louis J. Hampton, M.D., asked the Hanover Visiting Nurse Association to develop a respiratory home care program. The agency consented to start such a service.

To begin the program, the agency sent me—then a staff nurse—to Philadelphia for continuing education in comprehensive respiratory care. Soon after my return, we started the program, in 1969.

The first patient was a 24-year-old woman who had the facioscapulohumeral type of muscular dystrophy with secondary ventilatory insufficiency. She required tracheostomy care, assisted ventilation with a Bird respirator each night, postural drainage, chest physical therapy, and much emotional support. Her keenest wish was to remain at home and function adequately as a wife and mother. For four years, regular nursing visits helped her achieve this goal, although her physical condition continued to deteriorate.

During the same four years, the home care program grew steadily. The VNA periodically reviewed and revised policies, and it trained another nurse, Dawn Henry, as a respiratory specialist. She now directs the

BOBBY MALKUS, R.N., B.S.N., *is nurse director, Visiting Nurse Association, Hanover, Pa., and is a board member of the Pennsylvania Lung Association. As a staff nurse, she developed the program described here.*

respiratory home care program. In turn, she supervised the training of eight staff nurses in respiratory home care.

The VNA built up a large supply of equipment to lend, much of it through the generosity of individuals and service organizations. Families can rent or purchase equipment through the agency or the hospital's respiratory therapy department. A commercial supplier delivers oxygen to homes in the area.

When a patient is accepted for the home program, a respiratory care nurse makes the initial visit to determine the type and amount of care needed. The respiratory therapist from Hanover General Hospital accompanies the nurse on this visit, when his help is required.

One of our early patients, Edwin L., had asked his doctor to "do something before I die sitting here." He did not die sitting there, and we did "do something." His story illustrates what that "something" was.

A 65-year-old man with emphysema, Mr. L. had become increasingly incapacitated. He had not worked as a plasterer for two years. Shortness of breath interfered with even minimal personal hygiene, eating adequately, and lying down to sleep. He tried outpatient respiratory therapy for two months, but any benefits were nullified by the exhaustion that traveling to the hospital caused him.

His physician then hospitalized him for evaluation and treatment. Mr. L. was feeling apprehensive about his condition and future outlook, and an unfortunate incident elevated his anxiety to panic. One night when Mr. L. became short of breath, he requested something for relief. While the nurse was obtaining a medication order, he became confused, probably from cerebral anoxia. To protect him from injury, he was restrained in bed and his dentures removed.

By the time Mr. L.'s shortness of breath had been relieved, his panic was deep rooted and he was unable to respond positively to any therapy. He wished to go home, if only to die. At this point, the inhalation therapist and I agreed to try a home care program, although neither of us felt optimistic about its success.

On our first home visit, we found a large, two-story frame house in good repair. Ms. L., obese and tense, led us to a small, immaculate upstairs bedroom which was Mr. L.'s world. The room contained a bed, chest, and chair. There was a pleasant view of the backyard from the window.

Thin and gray, Mr. L. was sitting on the side of the bed, resting his head on his hands. He was markedly short of breath, his expression anxious. Ms. L. hovered at the door, her nervous mannerisms seeming to increase her husband's annoyance and anxiety. Both were apprehensive and indicated that they didn't believe home care would benefit Mr. L.

Our tentative respiratory rehabilitation plan specified daily IPPB treatments, chest physical therapy, postural drainage, and special attention to allay Mr. L's anxiety.

The respiratory therapist and I made the early home visits together, establishing rapport and building the couple's confidence in the possibility of improving life for them both. We included both Mr. and Ms. L. in planning, so they could regain some control over their situation. Detailed, repeated explanations of the disease process, plans for care, and procedures to be used were necessary.

We taught Mr. and Ms. L. to administer IPPB treatments with a rented, portable, Bird Mark 7 respirator four times daily, using 0.3 cc. isoproterenol (Isuprel) and 3 cc. saline. Mr. L. learned the positions for postural drainage and effective coughing. Ms. L. learned clapping and vibration. These procedures enabled Mr. L. to clear his chest of the copious, frothy secretions that collected constantly.

After the L.'s became easy about handling the equipment, I taught them to soak the nebulizing unit in a 1:3 solution of white vinegar and water, rinse it thoroughly, and air dry it. This routine proved satisfactory; Mr. L. has had no respiratory infections.

Because most patients showed anxiety when first placed on a home care program, I gave them my home telephone number and the respiratory therapist's, to use in an emergency. This service has never been abused. Mr. L., like other patients, called once or twice to be sure I was available. Then, feeling more secure, he did not use the emergency service.

Although Mr. and Ms. L. had modified their pattern of living, they needed assistance in making further rearrangments to conserve his energy. They found that, if Mr. L. bathed in the evening and prepared his clothing for the next day, he could manage with minimal shortness of breath. Organizing all bathing and shaving equipment on a roll-around kitchen cart, which Mr. L. pushed to the bathroom, was another suggestion that worked well.

As he improved enough to go downstairs, he carried his medication, pocket nebulizer, and other necessities in a light-weight basket. This also saved Ms. L. repeated trips up the stairs.

I taught Mr. L. controlled breathing, including diaphragmatic breathing and the pursed-lip maneuver, with practice and review at every visit until he mastered the techniques. To increase his exercise tolerance, I rigged a pulley in his doorway and taught him to exercise his arm, chest, and shoulder muscles.

He needed much encouragement. Ms. L. and I cooperated to encourage frequent exercise. After several weeks, Mr. L. began to discern muscle strengthening and increased exercise tolerance, an important step toward successful rehabilitation. For the first time, Mr. L. felt some hope. We added deep knee bends, and he progressed from one or two to a maximum of eight bends three times a day. He could now go downstairs for lunch and a short period. We gave him special training in controlled breathing while climbing stairs.

Mr. L. set the goal of walking outside by the time nice weather arrived, in about one month. Because he now recognized that exercise helped increase his activity tolerance, he agreed to work on an exercycle. The VNA loan closet provided one, and Mr. L. began his daily "rides to nowhere."

On the first warm spring day, Ms. L. and I accompanied a happy but somewhat apprehensive man for a 100-yard walk through his yard and back to the porch. Mr. L. had passed another important milestone.

By midspring, progress reached a plateau. Mr. L. now came downstairs daily for lunch and the afternoon. He could walk about a block and a half without discomfort on his good days and care for many personal needs. Mr. and Ms. L. seemed satisfied that he had come so far, but I believed he could progress further then he had.

I could find no reason for the halt until I discovered that Mr. L. watched a baseball game on TV each afternoon, and that to do this he had eliminated his afternoon exercise. We adjusted the daily schedule so that Mr. L. could have his prescribed exercise and his baseball game. I also instructed Mr. L. to walk about the house during commercial breaks and between innings to avoid prolonged inactivity.

Soon, we again noted slow progress. Activity goals were set, met, and reset. Mr. L. became able to drive his car to the grocery store, doctor's office, or his children's homes.

Because eating had increased his shortness of breath, Mr. L. often had refused to eat and had lost weight. Ms. L., a Pennsylvania Dutch woman, believed that "kissin' wears out, cookin' don't." Justly proud of her homemade cakes, pies, potpies, and other high caloric foods, she needed help to plan nourishing, light meals. She benefited personally from nutritional counseling, because she lost some weight. She learned to serve frequent small meals and to avoid gas-forming foods, which would result in pressure on the diaphragm and subsequent respiratory distress. Milk and milk products were limited, because they tend to thicken lung secretions. Mr. L. frequently took hot drinks like tea, coffee, bouillon, and drank six to eight glasses of water a day to keep secretions thin. In about eight months, his weight increased from 105 to 134 pounds, his optimum weight.

As Mr. L. progressed, I noticed restlessness and irritability, which seemed at first to be unreasonable. Ms. L. commented about this, for she felt Mr. L.'s attitude was straining their relationship. She thought they should be pleased with their accomplishments and satisfied with their quiet life.

One day following a visit by his daughter and her family. Mr. L. mentioned his loneliness. As we pursued this problem, Mr. L. talked at length about his sense of isolation and loss of social contact. He said that his friends avoided him, that he sensed that they thought he was malingering for he did not look sick. They could not understand the limitations that his constant shortness of breath imposed.

Following this discussion, I decided to proceed quickly with a project I had been considering. With the assistance of VNA staff, the hospital inhalation therapist, and the local lung association, I started an emphysema club. We began with 30 families. They enjoyed films, lectures, panel discussions, and social events. The opportunity to share experiences with others was an important benefit. Mr. and Ms. L. attended all sessions and enjoyed them thoroughly.

The club existed for three years and was then dropped due to dwindling attendance. Now, public education forums are offered periodically, instead.

Still another problem was financial. Mr. and Ms. L. worried a great deal about money. Mr. L. received a small pension from his employer and social security benefits. Although they owned their home, they had difficulty stretching their income to buy food, clothing, and medicine. Current and earlier medical bills had taken most of their savings. The VNA medical social worker helped them apply for Medicaid and food stamps and helped them learn to budget carefully.

Mr. L.'s pulmonary function and blood gas levels have not shown marked improvement, but he has learned to live a satisfying life within the limitations of his disease. The two are happy that his functioning has improved and that he has regained some independence. Together, they can cope with the problems emphysema has brought into their lives.

Mr. L. is one of the many people who have received care through the VNA's respiratory home care program. In 1974, 1,852 home visits were made to respiratory patients. In 1975, there were 1,927 nursing visits and 918 home health aide visits. We admitted 22 patients in 1975, and the respiratory therapist made 23 visits.

This program has prevented many readmissions to the hospital. It has helped patients and their families cope with respiratory disabilities and has showed the public that much can be done to assist people with chronic obstructive pulmonary disease.

From the *American Journal of Nursing* 76:416-418, Mar. 1976. Copyright © 1976. AJN Co.

Problems Families Face in Home Care

MARY ANN ROSE

Caring for the ill cancer patient and meeting family needs at the same time was one source of stress.

What goes on when a cancer patient is at home? Are home-care needs similar to or different from hospital-care needs? Is the emotional component in care more important or less important once the patient is home? Which community resources for assisting in care are acceptable in the home? What cultural influences affect home care?

The nurse may have personal experience to guide her in planning for the patient's discharge and there are nursing journal accounts of family disruption that may occur when a patient is at home(1,2,3). But there is no reported systematic study of the home-care needs of cancer patients or how they are met.

Because home care is assuming increasing importance as an alternative to costly institutional care, I reasoned that a study of home-care needs might aid nurses in discharge planning and aid members of community agencies in developing home-care programs.

I consulted the tumor registry of a large metropolitan hospital for the names of all cancer patients who had died between January and May 1973 and who lived at home sometime during the eight weeks preceding their deaths. I excluded anyone under 18 years of age at the time of death and anyone who had lived alone. Seventy-five families qualified for the study.

I wrote to the nearest relative of each patient who had died, asking if he or she would participate in the study. Approximately one third of the 75

MARY ANN ROSE, R.N., M.S.N., *is coordinator of clinical and community affairs, The Cancer Center, Cleveland, Ohio. This work was supported in part by the Cuyahoga County unit of the American Cancer Society.*

families could not be located even though only a few months had passed since the patient's death. Another one third of the families refused to participate for various reasons. This left one third, or 26 families, for interview.

In the questionnaire I designed, I asked about the patient's physical care and the family's social functioning while the ill person was at home. While the questionnaire did not include the word "cancer," it did use "tumor." No family members objected to this term.

Interviews ranged from 20 minutes to 3 hours. The relatives chose the place for the interview, usually the family home. I assured them that if they found the interview too difficult or painful I would not continue. Although many respondents wept, no one chose to stop.

What I learned was sometimes surprising, often poignant, and, on the whole, somewhat discouraging.

Most families reported that the patient's physical needs—such as bathing, feeding, and dressing changes—were met by immediate relatives or close friends. Only one of the 26 families reported that it had had visiting nurse assistance. It is difficult, therefore, to determine whether home nursing services would have made physical care easier for families.

Sixteen family members reported that they needed some type of special equipment to lighten the burden of the patient's physical care, but only 8 said that they obtained what they needed. Most items named as "needed but not obtained" were available locally, but I did not explore why families did not obtain the equipment.

Nineteen families indicated a need for teaching about home care, particularly in those areas requiring greater knowledge and judgment, such as pain control or special foods. Eleven received the suggestions they needed. For eight families, however, the teaching they received varied from none to some suggestions on how to give care or suggestions that were not helpful. I was unable to learn whether an attempt was made to teach the family during the patient's hospitalization, but, because of fatigue or anxiety, the family was unable to learn. Perhaps families were taught but could not transfer the learning to the home setting. If so, public health nurses might have helped families make the transition from hospital to home.

Almost all families reported that while the patient was at home, problems arose which they believed required a doctor's assistance. Fourteen families said that medical attention was inadequate. They wanted more information about the patient's status, help in giving injections, and help in coping with patient's "loss of manliness." Family members also looked to the physician as a primary source of emotional support on an ongoing basis.

Thirteen of the 26 family members mentioned problems in getting the patient to and from the hospital or clinic for treatment. Two major problems were the patient's need for physical support and the means of transportation. Two patients went to clinics by ambulance because they were unable to use conventional transportation. Eleven patients required the assistance of at least one other person. One woman reported that she had to quit her job because she was the only family member who could drive.

Three respondents spontaneously expressed their feelings about the last hospitalization. One stated that the family had sent the patient to the hospital to have a "quiet death." On the night of admission, many tests were taken. The patient was "treated poorly" in his last two hours, this respondent said, and he died in the x-ray department. Another reported that "mercy killing was done" because the patient died shortly after a medical procedure. But a third respondent said the hospital staff was kind and did "everything to help."

I found that family functions such as shopping and housekeeping continued during the time patients were at home. Assistance, when needed, came from within the extended family or from close friends. However, sleep, finances, and child care were identified as problems.

Twenty respondents reported difficulty in getting their usual amount of sleep. When asked why, seven replied that they were simply too worried to sleep. Two were afraid the patient would die, and one said that the patient snored, grumbled, or moaned all night. Another said that the patient would walk around at night, which awakened her. Providing care during the night was a reason for loss of sleep cited by 11 family members.

When asked if there were tasks that were troublesome to do because of their disrupted sleep, five respondents said yes. One woman replied that her cleaning was not done well. Another could not plan an evening out or shop regularly. One family member stated that she was unable to be on bed rest, which her doctor had ordered for her back problem, because of her care-giving responsibilities. Another respondent reported that he would have gone out to work during the day if he had not been up all night. He also commented that his wife, the patient, did not want him to leave her.

Two approaches could be used to help families get their sleep. Help in caring for the patient at night would allow family members to sleep. Many families did not go beyond the extended family or close friends for help with other problems, so one wonders whether the family would accept a stranger's presence at night. An alternate approach would be to provide day-time help so that the family could catch up on sleep. Each suggestion should be explored with families facing this problem.

I expected to find that cancer added another burden to family finances. While almost all families reported additional expenses, the financial disruption for most families was minimal. This may be because many patients were Medicare or Medicaid recipients. Four families, on the other hand, reported great disruption—they had to go on welfare because of the enormous expense, or they had to sell the house or property, or they were overwhelmed by unpaid bills. Here, financial counselors might have been part of the health team to advise the families about available community resources, for example, where equipment could be borrowed instead of purchased. These advisors could review insurance policies to assure that the families received all their benefits. They could also help patients make financial arrangements for the family after their death.

Only six families in my study had children at home. However, of these six, four reported problems in child care. This supports Issner's position that child care is difficult when one member of the family is hospitalized with a grave illness(4). However, a larger study than mine is necessary to determine whether the problems of caring for a cancer patient at home are more severe or different when there is a child in the home.

At the end of the interview, I asked family members for suggestions that "would help us plan more helpful services" for cancer patients. They replied at length, giving overwhelming support to the fact that caring for a cancer patient at home is a profound emotional burden.

They reported a sense of hopelessness about the diagnosis of cancer. Characteristic comments included "let the patient pretend he doesn't have cancer," "people should see a doctor more often so that cancer doesn't get a hold of you," and "what [services] can be helpful when you have cancer—none!"

The family members indicated that they expected the physician to give them emotional support and additional information rather than intervene to inhibit the progress of cancer or to cure it. In commenting on their emotional burdens, respondents mentioned the stress created by the wide range of demands in caring for the cancer patient along with maintaining the usual family functions.

In a general conversation at the end of the interview, they discussed talking to the patient about cancer or death. One person advised "never talk about cancer—keep up hope;" and another acknowledged that "telling her [the patient that she had cancer] was the hardest part." When she did tell the patient, she discovered that the patient had already arrived at this conclusion. Only one respondent advised that the family talk to the patient about dying, if possible.

And, finally, some respondents expressed concern that people do not know what a community offers. Others would have liked a nurse to visit, either to give care or to teach the family members how to give care. Some suggested that family counseling would have been helpful.

In reviewing my data, I found more questions than answers. I am hoping to replicate this study with a larger sample that includes families with children. In the whole area of home care, we have much to learn.

REFERENCES
1. BARCKLEY, VIRGINIA. The crisis in cancer. *Am. J. Nurs.* 67:278-280, Feb. 1967.
2. ISSNER, NATALIE. The family of the hospitalized child. *Nurs. Clin. North Am.* 7:5-12, Mar. 1972.
3. DRUMMOND, E. Impact of a father's illness. *Am. J. Nurs.* 64:89-91, Aug. 1964.
4. ISSNER, *op. cit.,* p.

From *Nursing Outlook* 23:574-577, Sept. 1975. Copyright © 1975. AJN Co.

Family Focus—
Transitional Health Care

KATHERINE F. SHEPARD • LOUISE M. BARSOTTI

In an attractive cottage on the hospital grounds, patients and their families learn to cope with problems that will confront them at home after the patient is discharged.

One summer morning in 1972, a Mexican-American family moved into a small cottage located 20 yards from one section of Stanford University Hospital Medical Center. One member of the family, a 62-year-old woman with recent bilateral below-knee amputations secondary to long-standing diabetes mellitus, was an inpatient at the medical center. With her was her husband, who spoke no English, and an 18-year-old niece, who acted as interpreter. This was the first family to take part in the Family Focus program, the hospital's pioneering transitional health care program for the inpatient in an acute care setting. Here, in this homelike setting, the patient and her family would experience what it would be like when she returned home.

That first night was a time of worry for the Family Focus staff. Would the patient and the family feel isolated? If something went wrong, would the switchboard operators initiate the emergency protocol effectively? How long would it take a nurse to reach the patient in the middle of the night?

During the course of the evening, the patient's family did place a call to the nursing supervisor—a request to have someone check a rash in the

MS. SHEPARD *(B.S., physical therapy, Ithaca College, N.Y.; M.A., physical therapy, Stanford University, Palo, Alto, Calif.) is instructor in the Division of Physical Therapy, Stanford University.* MS. BARSOTTI *(B.S., Stanford University School of Nursing) is administrative supervisor, Stanford University Hospital.*

patient's left axilla. The second, third, and fourth families that lived in Family Focus also called the nursing supervisor during their first evening in the cottage—and all for relatively minor complaints.

Then one day a staff member remarked, "I think the patient and family become frightened as night comes. They call to check out the system—to see if someone really is there." Thereupon the evening supervisor scheduled herself to make regular rounds at 9:00 P.M. on each family's first night of occupancy.

Since the schedule was acted on, there have been only two phone requests for aid at night from the 35 patients and their families who have subsequently lived in Family Focus. This was only one of many problems that arose and was solved during the implementation of this new type of health care.

OBJECTIVES OF PROGRAM

The Family Focus program was designed with two major objectives in mind. One was to determine the benefits of providing a time and a place *within* the hospital setting for a patient and his family to assume responsibility for the patient's health care—that is, to provide and evaluate a transitional health care experience. The second objective was to provide a setting in which to enhance the education of master's degree students in physical therapy by providing them with experiences related specifically to the social-behavioral aspects of illness and health.

Nursing, too, had an important role in this program. Although the Family Focus program was designed by faculty at the Division of Physical Therapy at Stanford University Medical Center, in collaboration with psychologists from the Mental Research Institute in Palo Alto, it has become a reality primarily through the cooperation and support of the nursing service and members of the other allied health professions at Stanford University Hospital.

THE SETTING

The setting for Family Focus is a small, prefabricated building containing a bedroom, bathroom, living room, dining room/family room, and kitchen. There are convertible couches in both the living and family room areas so that a total of six family members can be accommodated. Second-hand furnishings give the house a warm, lived-in, home-like quality.

Only a limited number of modifications for disabled patients have been built into the house, and the adaptations that are included, such as a lever-like handle on the kitchen faucet for patients who have insufficient hand grasp to turn a faucet handle, may be purchased in any local hardware store. In the bedroom, the patient sleeps in a standard-size single bed, and in the bathroom an ordinary wooden chair is used for a bathtub seat. One small section of the building has been set aside as a base of operation for the Family Focus staff.

TYPES OF PATIENTS

There are few specific criteria for the types of patients who can be involved in the Family Focus program. To qualify, the patient must be referred by his attending physician; he must be receiving physical therapy at the time of admission to Family Focus; and he and his family must live within approximately 50 miles of Stanford University Medical Center.

To date, the patients have ranged in age from four months to 92 years, with such diverse diagnoses as cardiovascular accidents, total hip replacements, heart transplants, and carcinoma. The patient's "family" who will accompany him into Family Focus might include a spouse, children, other relatives, friends, or a housekeeper—even family pets. For safety reasons, the family must include at least one responsible adult.

PERSONNEL INVOLVED

Patients, along with their families, move into Family Focus for the last three days of their inpatient hospital stay. During this time the hospital staff works with the patient and family members to teach them the rehabilitative and preventive health care skills they will need to care for the patient at home.

On any one day, in addition to intensive work with the physical therapist, the patient and family may be visited by the dietitian (to discuss the preparation of food for the patient's special dietary needs), the occupational therapist (to help the family consider adaptive equipment), and/or the social worker (to counsel on financial planning).

Of course, members of the nursing staff assigned to the patient and his family visit regularly each day. The nurse functions primarily as a public health nurse might when making a home visit. She teaches the patient and the family any required nursing skills, observes return demonstrations, and ascertains further nursing needs. One day-shift nurse is defined as the primary person responsible for the nursing care activity during the family's three-day stay. She is assisted, as needed, by the supervisors.

In attempting to formulate a program responsive to the philosophy of transitional care in acute care settings, many program possibilities were considered. These ranged from a one-day stay by a member of the patient's family to a family live-in period of a week or more for those patients who had considerable permanent physical disabilities.

To have a patient and family involved in at least one overnight stay was considered imperative, since it was during this 24-hour period that many problems concerning care of the patient arise. For example, additional family stress is evidenced when a patient needs to be assisted with toileting or repositioning several times during the night. Experience has shown that such stress on a spouse or another member of the family has been enough to severely disrupt the family structure.

A two-night stay was found to be the optimal time span. It was long enough for the family to discover the need for, learn, and practice new skills and to feel sufficiently at ease to ask questions frankly of the health care personnel.

PROBLEMS AND SOLUTIONS

Other problems have arisen simply in terms of the physical setting of the Family Focus unit. For example, where should the patient's chart be kept? Should nursing supplies be kept in the cottage if the latter is supposed to replicate as nearly as possible the patient's own home setting? What sort of call system should be established between the family's living quarters and the nearest nursing station?

These problems were solved primarily by trial and error and by holding as close as possible to the established protocol for traditional nursing unit setups within the hospital. For example, the patient's chart is kept in the Family Focus staff area during the day. At 5:00 P.M. it is returned to the nearest nursing unit, where it is available for the night supervisory staff or physicians in case there should be an emergency during the night.

It was decided not to keep additional nursing equipment in the house, as this would distort the homelike setting and make the patient and family feel more dependent on the hospital.

The call system is set up with the name of the assigned nurse and her telephone number posted on the wall by the family's telephone. If the needs of the family and patient are more than their assigned day-shift nurse can take care of, they are instructed to call the switchboard operator and ask for the evening or night supervisor.

THE FIRST DAY

For the first 24 hours or so in Family Focus, the patient and his family behave much like anyone moving into a new setting for the first time—for example, like a student moving into a college dormitory at the beginning of the fall quarter. They tend to be somewhat subdued; there is a great deal of investigation and rearrangement of the physical environment and an atmosphere of apprehension as they wait to see which health care personnel will appear next.

However, after the first night, the patient and family begin to act in a progressively self-determined and even aggressive manner. They seem to settle down into a pattern of interaction with one another much as they would at home. Conflicts, apprehensions, and humor come to the fore easily. The hospital personnel are treated as guests who enter the family's home.

Patients and family members become very specific in designating those areas of health care that they need assistance with. Perhaps a bathtub transfer has been tried and failed, and so they ask for assistance on a better method. Or they may be confused about medication and ask for help in setting up an effective time system, or they want to be shown how to crush a pill.

A STRIKING DIFFERENCE

The most striking difference between the patients and families in this transitional setting and those in the traditional inpatient care setting is that the Family Focus patients prove to be much more psychologically resilient and physically capable when the members of their families form a familiar support system around them. Patients who have needed several members of the nursing staff to help them move from a bed to a wheelchair on the traditional hospital unit, for example, are often able to do the same transfer with only a single family member.

Explanations for this ability might include the fact that the patient receives timely instructions, has repeated practice sessions, an increased sense of responsibility for himself, and a family-supported desire to succeed.

In turn, the hospital staff respond to the patient's health care needs, as defined collaboratively with the patient and his family, rather than designating unilaterally what these needs might be. Time and again, patients and families have not only shown themselves to be realistic and capable in the definition of their health care needs but have also given the hospital personnel tremendous insight into how patients and families experience and subsequently adapt to these needs in their own unique life style.

The psychologists on the Family Focus staff provide continuous consultation—not to patients and family members, but to the health care personnel involved with them. The emphasis has been on teaching personnel how to observe and understand patient-family interactions, how to identify the intervention techniques most useful for teaching families, and how to prepare the patient and family for the psychosocial as well as physical adjustments they will need to make.

THE MAIN DIFFICULTY

The main difficulty encountered by the nursing personnel assigned to the Family Focus unit has been, as in the traditional setting, the problem of time. Although the nurse gives the family only an average of three hours for a three-day stay—rather than four to eight hours a day as in a traditional setting—nearly all of that time is provided by a single nurse. Additionally, she must care for a group of inpatients.

She has found that she needs time, too, to "switch gears" into the role she assumes with her Family Focus patients and families. What often happens is that the nurse quickly becomes caught up with the problems and needs of the patients and families and stays beyond her traditional work day to discuss and help implement the suggestions she had made for alleviating problems.

In a poll taken for the first ten nurses assigned for Family Focus, 70 percent of them said the greatest advantage of working in that setting is that they come to understand the philosophy and utility of health care given within a context of a family unit, rather than a patient unit. They reported that the experience had helped them make better use of discharge planning with their in-hospital patients.

There is probably no better place than Family Focus to observe the health care team in action. The following is an example.

Mrs. B has moved into the Family Focus cottage with her husband. Between them, this elderly couple has suffered a long list of physical disabilities, ranging from partial loss of sight, loss of upright balance, low walking endurance, and some degree of cognitive senility. In the estimation of the hospital staff during the time the patient was in the hospital, there was no way in which she and her equally disabled husband could manage at home alone.

However, the couple were adamant; they wanted to return home, and they wanted the Family Focus experience. And so it was arranged for them. A large part of the couple's problem was medication. Neither the husband nor the patient, individually, could remember times, dosages, and types of medication.

After several attempts, the nurse and the physical therapist worked out a system whereby the husband, under the guidance of a next-door neighbor, would lay out the weekly allotment of medications in an empty egg carton. The wife, who could not remember the type or dosage, could remember the times for the medication. Together, they resolved the problem. Follow-up after three months showed the medication system working effectively and the couple thriving.

By working with the family and the patient in the Family Focus setting, the nursing staff, physical therapist, physicians, and other members of the health care team have learned to work together in a manner responsive to the patient and family health care needs that is difficult to conceive of and achieve in an in-hospital setting.

Section V Alternative Settings for Community Health Nursing Practice

A variety of community settings in which nurses are practicing are described in this section, including physician offices, jails, industry, specialty clinics, camps, and health maintenance organizations. The special demands of each of these settings call upon the nurse to devise strategies to deal with the responsibilities involved and techniques to deliver health care services.

From the *American Journal of Nursing* 75:442-445, Mar. 1975. Copyright © 1975. AJN Co.

Office Nursing in a Problem-Oriented Practice

JANETTE E. TAYLOR

A nurse traces the job that evolved in unusual ways over a decade.

If someone had told me 10 years ago when I first came to work as an office nurse in a two-man practice what I would be doing now, I'm not sure that I would have had the courage or the confidence to take the position.

It seemed simple enough then. In fact, I was mostly receptionist and secretary, insurance clerk and bookkeeper in those days. But the practice was unique; for five years, it had used the then new problem-oriented system(1). At that time, however, the problem-oriented system was a simple method of listing problems by number and title, organizing the information into subjective and objective findings, and designing a plan for action for each problem(2).

The system and I have done a lot of growing and changing since then. I find it impossible to discuss what I do out of the context of the problem-oriented system, since my work, as well as that of everyone in the office from receptionist to physician, is so thoroughly intertwined with it.

When difficulties arise, we have to see if these are problems of the system itself or of performance within the system. It is evaluation of this type (audit) which has enabled the system to change from a simple

MS. TAYLOR, R.N., *after years of being professionally inactive, returned to nursing in the Promis Clinic, Hampden Highlands, Me. Promis is a private clinic that has become nationally known for its leadership in the problem-oriented medical system, in the development and use of protocols for various diseases, and for the kind of communication system maintained between health professionals and their consumers.*

form of record keeping to a sophisticated system of health care, capable of using nonphysicians at all levels, when given defined guidelines for performance, to deliver quality health care.

My formal education consists of a three-year hospital-based nursing program. The rest of my education has been on an individual person-to-person basis with physicians, patients, and others along the way—perhaps the first and most basic being my mother, who had a lot of old-fashioned common sense, some of which I assimilated. I also believe that the life experiences of having raised a family of five children and having worked through several family crises give me some credibility and insight with patients.

My early experience in this practice was more clerical than clinical, and this was probably good. The older nurse who has been profession-

---

ASHD, Without Failure

RN Management Protocol

CRITERIA: Recent myocardial infarction, episode of coronary insufficiency (pain lasting 10-20 min), typical angina.

GOALS: Post MI—to return to useful function within 6-8 wks. of event, either in previous job or another via rehabilitation and retraining;
Angina—to attain highest level of function, both vocationally and in personal life with minimum of pain;
All—to detect and treat early major complications—recurrent infarction, arrhythmia, congestive failure, depressive/adjustment reaction, arterial embolism, bleeding (if on anticoagulant therapy).

RECORD:
S: *New* breathlessness, chest pain, PND, ankle swelling. On patients with angina—amount of pain (av. ≠ NTG/day), relation to physical activity, sleep, emotional upset, eating, sexual activity and duration and relief with NTG.
O: Weight, apical pulse (listen for 1 min), BP—each visit. Peak flow if patient reports new or changed symptoms.
A: Discuss progress, changes in Rx and reasons. Explain any factors limiting control, such as another concurrent problem, poor patient cooperation, environmental, etc.
P: *More data*—ECG lead II if new, >5, premature beats. Full ECG if chest pain lasts more than 20 min, unrelieved by NTG. For patients on Coumadin, protime at weekly intervals until stable within 5 sec, then at intervals to be specified by doctor. Chest X-ray for heart size 3 mos. post-MI.
Therapy—1. Weight control/diet. Attempt to maintain ideal weight. Restrict animal fats, dairy fats. No salt added. Limit coffee to <5 cups/day.
2. Reduce or eliminate *cigarette smoking*—pipe/cigar ok if not inhaled.
3. Exercise/Activity: Post-MI—to be outlined by physician. Angina—program outlined in Post Graduate Medicine, 9/70, p 219. Gradual increase in walking to 2-3 miles/day at rate of 15 min/mi, or by using exercycle for equal distance.

ally inactive sometimes feels that medical technology has gone so far that she cannot or will not devote the time and energy for formal refresher courses to catch up. Using the problem-oriented system and protocols for management, she will learn while doing. In transcribing the problem-oriented dictation, I was learning what symptoms are peculiar to particular problems, what parameters are monitored and why, and how to follow the doctor's analysis.

As receptionist, I quickly became aware of how different ambulatory care is from hospital care. To be able to identify which patients needed to be seen immediately and which needed comprehensive exams but not urgently, I had to learn what problems we couldn't afford to miss and what screening questions identified potentially dangerous situations. I learned to reassure anxious mothers, to recognize panic and get the

---

4. Drugs: a) NTG grs. 1/150 (1/100, 1/200), sublingually *PRN* up to 10/day. Caution re dizziness/lightheadedness (infrequent) within 3-5 min. after use. Inform *re* headache/pounding immediately after taking med or burning sensation under the tongue indicates drug is still potent and is a common side effect. Inform *re* losing potency after 3 mos. even though med kept in dark, tightly covered container. Instruct patients in prophylactic use, before entering into activity previously found to cause pain. (Write Rx for = 100 and dispense in original bottle).

b) *Isosorbide Dinitrate* (Isordil) 5-10 mg. sublingually after meals and hs. Try if angina occurs more than twice daily. May use Tembids, 40 mg. bid, long acting. Use in conjunction with NTG.

c) *Propanolol* (Inderal) 10 and 40 mg. tabs. Start 10 mg. q4h when awake, and increase by 10 mg/dose until symptoms controlled and pulse maintained >50 and < 70 or total dose of 150 mg/day reached. May be used on patients still having angina on drugs in (a) and (b). Contraindicated in CHF, asthma, COPD.

d) *Warfarin* (Coumadin)—use after hospital phase of acute MI. Use in preinfarction angina controversial. When used, physician must state rationale, documentation and program for following. Physician must also state duration of treatment.

Pt. Educ—Amer. Heart Assn booklets "After a Heart Attack" and/or "Angina". Give copy of flow sheet. Emphasize patient must do the work. Stress importance of reporting *immediately* new/increasing frequency of chest pain.

REFER and/or *CONSULT* PHYSICIAN:

Sx: New/increased chest pain,↑SOB, sx not covered by protocol, ankle swelling, PND.

O: New elevation BP >160/95, systolic <100, P>100 or <50, PVC's >5/min, wgt. gain 1 lb. per week x 4 weeks, new edema >1+, ↓ peak flow by 15%. Pro time · 20 sec on Coumadin. BUN >30, uric acid 9.0.

PT.ED: Poor reliability (missed appointments, not taking meds, etc.). Wants to see doctor. For yearly physical.

Ref. Epstein, S.E., Redwood R.E., et al. Angina pectoris, pathophysiology, evaluation and treatment. *Ann. Int. Med.* 75, 263, 1971.

Ms. Taylor helped develop this and other protocols for chronic conditions.

patient to some help, and to face an occasional irate, sometimes irrational, patient.

I helped to develop the first automated histories we used and worked on subsequent revisions, when we asked, "Is this question really necessary" thereby cutting the bulk of the questionnaire. The doctors had been making individual flow sheets for the persons whose problems gave them many parameters to follow, but as the practice grew, they didn't have time to do this. I helped design flow sheets for common diseases—cardiovascular diseases, diabetes, chronic lung disease, and, later on, for life problems and arthritis.

On the back of the flow sheet are listed the usual medications for that specific disease group, along with dosage, relative contraindications, symptomatic side effects, and monitoring information. Again, helping with the development of these was a learning experience for me, and through it all, the doctors were evaluating my behavioral traits of reliability, efficiency, analytic sense, and thoroughness.

Concurrently, I learned lab skills—venipunctures, complete blood counts, urinalysis, blood sugars, sedimentation rates, cultures—and some of the physiologic testing. I learned to test reflexes, listen for breath sounds and carotid bruits, and test pulmonary function and ocular tension, among others.

Then in middle 1970, the decision was made to let me do some of the follow-up care on long-term patients. These would be patients who had had their initial comprehensive evaluation by the physician, who had developed a complete problem list with plans for treatment of each problem. Those who were referred to me had chronic problems that needed to be monitored regularly. At first, I saw the patient assigned, gathered the information I thought to be pertinent, and then called the doctor in. We reviewed the data and discussed the continuing treatment.

By January 1971, a set of protocols for the treatment of arteriosclerotic heart disease, chronic lung disease, diabetes, peripheral vascular disease, obesity, anxiety, conversion, and depression had been developed. These were joint efforts by the physicians and me. At that time, I started seeing the patients on my own, only calling in the physician when needed. The protocols listed criteria for diagnoses, overall goals, the minimal subjective and objective information, diagnostic and therapeutic plans, and patient education as well as criteria for referral (one being whether the patient *wanted* to see the doctor that day).

EARLY EXPERIENCES

In the beginning I was quite uneasy and unsure of myself. Many of those assigned to me were elderly, and when I realized that mostly they needed understanding and education and caring, my job became much easier. Many times, they expressed their appreciation for my taking the time to answer their questions, which they felt were "too stupid" to ask the doctor. We found, often, that the patients were much too nervous to remember what the doctor had told them. If they remembered one thing, they were doing well.

Several times on follow-up I found that they had taken the medication ordered till it was gone, but then didn't get a refill. By the time I saw them, they may have been out of medication for several days—"didn't want to get a refill since I might not have to take it any more." I found that particularly on their first visit with me, it was helpful to review all the plans for therapy to be sure the patient understood them.

Currently, since the patient does receive a copy of the doctor's dictated note of the comprehensive evaluation, this is not so critical, although some still do not understand what they are to do with it. Our patients all receive summaries of their present health care status with a covering letter asking them to audit the summary for accuracy and to make any additions and corrections and to indicate whether they understand the care plans. If they wish, their entire medical record is made available to them, with a small charge for reproducing the entire chart of raw data.

I type my own notes of each visit—problem oriented, of course—so that whoever sees the patient next time will know what is going on, what the patient has been told, and what is expected of the patient. If I should not be available when the patient needs care, any one of the physicians at the clinic could as easily see him.

I see my role as primarily educational. When a patient has a diagnosis made—hypertension, diabetes, obesity, whatever—he wants and needs to know what he can do about it, what he can expect to happen, what effect this will have on his daily life, and how he can adjust. The patient not only is given a copy of his physical note, but may also have a copy of the flow sheet. This is a good tool to use, for the more you can get the patient to accept the responsibility for his own care, the better his compliance in the treatment program will be.

Let's just look at a 45-year-old man, 20 pounds overweight, blood pressure 170/100 on three determinations, cholesterol and triglycerides of 320 and 289 respectively, with a Lipoprotein pattern, phenotype IV. He smokes one to two packs of cigarettes a day. He used to be quite active physically, but now is a salesman on the road a lot and eats many meals out. The business he is in is pressured. There is a lot of competition.

He is so tired when he gets home at night that he has no desire to do anything but plop down in front of the TV. His wife is concerned. She is involved in several community activities but he is always "too tired" to go with her. His teenagers are pretty good kids, he feels, but he can't seem to talk to them, much less understand them, so he ignores them. He feels quite frustrated.

GOAL SETTING

Obviously, there are many things here to consider and I have to decide what one or two things will make the most impact. After talking a bit about risk factors, we can together set some short-term goals (overall goals were set at the time of his comprehensive evaluation).

I will give him a Type IV American Heart Association diet without added salt, as a guideline, and outline with him some sort of regular exercise program. Perhaps he can park his car several blocks from his office or where he has an appointment and walk briskly those blocks, increasing the distance gradually. Maybe he can get involved in a Y program. This probably would be all I would get into on the first visit, and I would give him a month to see how he would implement this treatment regimen.

At the second visit, he has been walking faithfully and trying to stick to his diet. The increased exercise has given him more energy; he's sleeping better and walking off some of his tensions. He has started golfing with his son and finds that they do have things they can talk about. He has even gone to a couple of community/church activities with his wife, and there are some people he would like to know better. And wonder of wonders, his sex drive is stronger; he'd begun to think he was "over the hill," but "of course, couldn't talk to anyone about that."

His weight has dropped only three pounds, but his muscles are tightened up some. He notes that his pants are looser and he has had to take in his belt one notch. His blood pressure today is 160/95, an acceptable level. He can be shown the change on the graphic sheet.

He feels much better, and therein lies a danger; he may start to backslide. Support does need to be continued and he needs to be told the statistics on the relationship of smoking to circulation and cardiovascular disease.

In six months, his blood lipids are normal, his weight is normal, his blood pressure continues to be within normal limits, and he is sleeping well and has plenty of energy. He is still working on the smoking, but, in general, he feels great.

Obviously, this is a well-motivated guy. Results are not always this dramatic, but sometimes significant results come from relatively small changes. You must look at the whole picture, set priorities, see what one or two changes will set off the greatest chain reaction, and then throw your whole effort into helping the patient change that behavior which will affect his health.

Sometimes the patient's relationships with his family or co-workers have gone awry. This is reflected in physical symptoms for which the physician can find no physiologic basis. When these persons are referred to me for counseling, I find that using transactional analysis techniques is helpful(3). Generally, these people have a poor self-image. They feel not-OK most of the time and may cover up their feelings by overreacting (overeating, oversmoking, overdrinking, and so forth).

This is particularly true of grossly obese patients. Their poor self-concept is reinforced every time they go by a mirror or a store window, or try to buy clothes, or exercise—just about anything. Even if they do lose 15 to 20 pounds by conscientious dieting, it hardly shows, so they get depressed, and the vicious circle is completed, for depression is often one reason for compulsive eating.

It has been suggested that followup or chronic care may be very humdrum and uninteresting. I have not found it so. When I look at a chronic problem in the light of the patient's total problem list, each patient becomes different, because of the different set of circumstances involved. This is still a learning situation. When it ceases to be, then I will know I am ready to retire!

INDEPENDENCE—COLLABORATION

Using the problem-oriented system and defined protocols, the nurse can work independently, yet closely in cooperation with the physician, in providing quality health care. I have learned to structure my thinking as I write progress notes in the prescribed SOAP (Subjective, Objective, Assessment, Plan-diagnostic, therapeutic, and patient education) fashion, looking at each problem in the light of the total problem list. This then makes the record easy to follow, easy to audit, for me as well as others, to see if plans have been carried out, if goals are being accomplished. This feedback loop then furnishes material for education of both the patient and the professional persons who are supervising his care. I am free to work within our general guidelines in a manner tailored to each patient as I see his needs.

REFERENCES

1. BJORN, J. C., AND CROSS, H. D. *Problem Oriented Practice.* Chicago, Modern Hospital Press, 1970.
2. HURST, J. W., AND WALKER, H. K., EDS. *The Problem Oriented System.* New York, MEDCOM, 1972.
3. HARRIS, T. A. *I'm OK, You're OK.* New York, Harper & Row, 1967.

From the *American Journal of Nursing* 76:95-97, Jan. 1976. Copyright © 1976. AJN Co.

Improving Health Care for Troubled Youths

JANET GARZONE KOSIDLAK

An expanded health program and the establishment of a full-time nursing position were the results of a nurse's survey of the health problems of 296 persons, aged eight to seventeen, detained at a juvenile center.

Detention is one of the most common means by which American society tries to solve many social and criminal problems. A person may be detained before trial, and/or after trial. The child or adolescent usually is detained in a juvenile center or court-assigned home; the adult, in a prison or jail.

Studies of the literature by social scientists, penologists, and health researchers suggest that the incidence of ill health, both physical and mental, is much greater in any detainee group than in the general population(1). Yet, in spite of wide recognition that the physical, mental, and social problems of troubled children are interrelated, the court rarely benefits from the knowledge, skill, or research potential of the relevant fields of science(2).

In Norfolk, Virginia, the jail is the responsibility of the police department, while the prison farm and youth detention center are managed by the Norfolk Department of Human Resources. Traditionally, both adult and juvenile detainees have received limited health care from a contract physician for episodic care, a detention center staff member

JANET GARZONE KOSIDLAK, R.N., M.S., *is director of nursing, Department of Public Health, Newport News Health Center, Newport News, Va. The program she describes took place under her supervision as director of nursing services in the Norfolk Health Department, Va.*

acting as a "medic," and the Norfolk Public Health Department as a back-up in the special crises of such illnesses as venereal disease and tuberculosis. Certain obvious inadequacies result from such a program of care.

An opportunity for the Norfolk Health Department (NHD) to intervene in the health program for juvenile detainees arose in February 1972 when the director of the youth center asked the NHD to provide a temporary nurse to replace the center's parttime nurse, who had resigned, and to evaluate the need for a full-time nurse. Supervisory personnel at the youth center, who were carrying out the activities of the nurse who had resigned, had complained that they were neither qualified nor competent to make decisions about the detainees' health care.

The NHD assigned a public health nurse to provide episodic care at the center from 2:00 to 4:00 P.M., Monday through Friday, and to be available for consultation from 8:00 A.M. to 2:00 P.M. each day. This resolved the immediate staffing crisis.

The medical and nursing staff of the NHD then explored the desirability of expanding the health care offered to the youths in detention. Records at the youth center revealed that most nursing services had been related to the episodic illnesses of the children. The former parttime nurse, employed four hours daily, Monday through Friday, had assessed their physical complaints at sick call or on demand, decided whether medical care was needed immediately or could be deferred until the physician's next visit, and had telephoned the physician in emergencies or for special information. For routine communication, the nurse had used the clinic log to record the date and time, the youth's name and complaint, and the assessment of illness, treatment, and his or her proposed disposition.

Barring an emergency, the physician had visited the youth center three times weekly at varying hours, depending on the demands of his private practice. After sick call, the physician wrote his orders in the clinic log and returned to his practice.

The next step was a seven-month survey by the public health nurse at the youth center of the sequential health records of all 296 youths who were detained between March 1 and September 25, 1972. Of these adolescents, 34 percent were female, 66 percent were male. One percent was between the ages of 8 and 11, 39 percent between 12 and 14, and 56 percent between 16 and 17. The number of black and white youths who were detained was the same.

The nurse identified 331 health problems among the 296 detainees.

HEALTH PROBLEMS OF 296 DETAINEES AGED 8 TO 17 YEARS

Problem	Number	Not treated, not referred
• Breast mass	1	0
• Convulsions	1	0
• Disorders affecting the following:		
ears	3	2
eyes	31	31
heart	9	9
musculoskeletal system (shoulder deformity)	1	1
nose	5	4
skin	75	61
teeth	88	74
throat	33	11
• Drug abuse, admitted or suspected	4	3
• Emotional/mental disorders (other than sleeping disturbances)	18	0
• Family planning (IUD or pills used prior to detention)	11	7 (method not continued during detention)
• Hernia	1	1
• Obesity	17	17
• Pregnancy	12	1 confirmed by lab test / 11 unconfirmed
• Undernutrition	5	5
• Venereal disease, suspected	16	0
Total	331*	238

*Total exceeds 296 because some youths had more than one health problem.

A total of 248 health problems remained untreated and had not been referred to community resources by the end of the youths' confinement.

To collect these data, the public health nurse interviewed and evaluated each youth on the day of admission to the center, and recorded her findings on a standard health examination record. The nurse's assessment consisted of a short history of past acute and recurring illnesses, communicable diseases, allergies, operations, hospitalizations, immunizations, and behavioral aberrations. The physical inspection included general appearance, height, weight, blood pressure, vision and hearing screening, examination of throat, teeth, skin, posture, and gait.

Laboratory study consisted of urinalysis for sugar and acetone.

All health care intervention during the youth's detention at the center was recorded on a standard health examination review. This provided a complete, chronological account of each youth's initial evaluation, episodic illnesses, treatment, and outcomes.

The survey findings (summarized in the box) indicated the need for a more adequate episodic and emergency treatment program at the Youth Detention Center, for improved physical and emotional health services, for preventive and health educational services, and for the referral of youths for continuing health care after their release. The data demonstrated the need to obtain special medical assistance for the venereal disease, obstetrical, family planning, and surgical problems of the youths.

The survey data replicated the conclusion in a study of 255 "healthy" females attending a contraceptive clinic in New York City that "the female teenager considered to be at the healthiest time of life is in reality not without significant pathology"(3).

It was impossible to classify the 331 health problems as distinctly physical, emotional, or social because the etiology of many of these problems is probably a combination of all three. Obesity certainly has physical, emotional, and socioeconomic causes, and it may be assumed that other problems also have multiple causes.

A final report including the following four recommendations was presented to the directors of health, personnel, and budget:

• physical examination of each youth by a physician or nurse practitioner in order to detect new illness, assess the current status and management of chronic illness, and thus begin treatment of newly diagnosed conditions on the youth's admission or continue treatment of his chronic conditions without interruption during the period of detention.

• standing orders for laboratory tests for anemia, pregnancy, urinary tract infections, and venereal disease, so that, with early laboratory confirmation, treatment can be initiated promptly.

• a full-time public health nurse position at the youth center under the supervision of the Norfolk Health Department. (As an NHD staff member the nurse would receive health-oriented rather than correction-oriented direction and supervision; have access to the NHD records of the many children and their families known to the health department through school health, crippled child, child health, family planning, tuberculosis, and venereal disease programs; and have available the educational and consultant programs of the Bureau of Nursing of the State Department of Health.)

- a role description for the public health nurse who is to practice at the youth center, in terms of seven specific functions:

1. assessing every child for developmental aberrations, impaired sight and hearing, physical defects, injuries, possible drug abuse, nutrition, communicable disease, and acute and long-term illnesses
2. obtaining pertinent health information from other community agencies
3. developing and coordinating a comprehensive plan of health care with the physician, youth center staff, and parents
4. communicating the plan of health care to the juvenile court to assure provision of continuity of care
5. establishing teaching sessions on family life, nutrition, pregnancy, handling stress, care of the skin to alleviate acne and other conditions common to youths, drug abuse, and venereal disease
6. providing individual and group counseling for youths who have emotional disorders
7. teaching youth center supervisors to give oral medications and to do minor treatments and teaching that would include first aid principles and the side effects of drugs.

ACTION AND RESULTS

The recommendations were accepted with one modification, and a full-time nurse was hired in late 1973. The nurse was appointed to the youth center staff instead of the NHD staff because the city could obtain 90 percent federal funding for center positions while the NHD could obtain only 55 percent funding. The advantage of the relationship between the NHD and the center was appreciated, however, and the public health nurse who had been working temporarily at the center became the liaison person among the new full-time nurse at the center, the health department, and other community agencies.

Using the nursing process, the nurse obtained a data base of each youth's past health history, current status, and use of primary health care and community resources. The nurse then assessed the child for developmental aberrations, impaired sight and hearing, physical defects, injuries, possible drug abuse, communicable diseases, illnesses, and nutritional status.

The goals for the care of the youths, formulated from the initial data base, were to complete the data base by an interview with the child's parent or guardian, to initiate medical referral for chronic and acute conditions, to correct defects, and to provide health education, counseling, and continuity of care. A care plan was formulated and services to correct problems were begun.

Medical care was provided through a cooperative effort of the physician at the Youth Detention Center, the primary care physician (private or clinic), the specialist (private or clinic), and the local and state programs.

After six months, the program was reviewed. This initial evaluation showed that youthful detainees were receiving more continuous care from a full-time health professional but that comprehensive care for all detainees was still to be achieved.

The activities of the nurse at the youth center had increased gradually as she became more knowledgeable in history taking, child assessment, and use of community resources, and more adept in direct intervention. The liaison functions of the public health nurse had decreased as she helped the resident nurse become more self-sufficient, and had changed to consultation.

An important accomplishment was that the correctional staff recognized the value of continuing the new health care program at the youth center. A summary report of each child's health record, health recommendations, and care plan was included with the mittemus (court sheet).

The development of health services has been based on the "Health Standards for Juvenile Court Residential Facilities" of the American Academy of Pediatrics Committee for Youth. This committee recognizes that youths in detention centers display a high incidence of physical and mental health problems due to inadequate care and nurturing in the past(1).

In 1973 the mayor appointed a Human Resources Council with representatives from the departments of health, planning, and human resources. Matters pertinent to juvenile detention are brought to the council for joint consideration.

Health services to troubled youths continue to improve and the academy's standards remain the blue print for these services.

REFERENCES

1. AMERICAN ACADEMY OF PEDIATRICS, COMMITTEE ON YOUTH. Health standards for juvenile court residential facilities. *Pediatrics 52:452-457, Sept. 1973.*
2. POTIER, WISE. The child and the law—contemporary situation in juvenile justice. *Am. J. Public Health* 63:386-389, May 1973.
3. FIEDLER, D. E., AND OTHERS. Pathology in the "healthy" female teenager. *Am. J. Public Health* 63:962-965, Nov. 1973.

From the *American Journal of Nursing* 75:1755-1760, Oct. 1975. Copyright © 1975. AJN Co.

The Quality of the Work Environment

MARY LOUISE BROWN

> *Occupational health is an important aspect of the total health care system. One protective aspect of that system is the Occupational Safety and Health Act which seeks to preserve our human resources by controlling job hazards.*

The quality of the environment in which we live and work is a vital issue. Advances in technology and the increased use of chemicals have caused our life support systems to become so polluted that our very survival is endangered.

The federal government's involvement in pollution control has been expressed in a series of acts: the Air Quality Act of 1955, the Solid Waste Disposal Act of 1965, a second Air Quality Act in 1967, the Federal Coal Mine Health and Safety Act of 1969, and the Occupational Safety and Health Act of 1970. The concerns expressed by the Congress in the environment in which people work are concerns for human health and, therefore, the Occupational Safety and Health Act of 1970 obviously has specific implications for nursing.

When Congress enacted Public Law 91-596—the Occupational Safety and Health Act—it declared as its purpose: "to assure so far as possible every working man and woman in the Nation safe and healthful working conditions and to preserve our human resources"(1). This goal was to be accomplished by encouraging employers and employees to reduce the number of safety and health hazards in workplaces, and by stimu-

MARY LOUISE BROWN, R.N., M.A., *is regional program director, P.H.S. Region II, National Institute for Occupational Safety and Health and a knowledgeable, experienced occupational health nurse.*

lating employers and employees to develop new or to perfect existing programs for providing safe and healthful working conditions.

The Act created three federal agencies: the National Institute for Occupational Safety and Health, or NIOSH, in the U.S. Department of Health, Education, and Welfare; the Occupational Safety and Health Administration, or OSHA, in the U.S. Department of Labor; and the Occupational Safety and Health Review Commission, an independent agency to carry out the adjudicatory functions.

NIOSH functions as the principal federal agency engaged in research on the health effects of job hazards. It is responsible for identifying occupational safety and health hazards and for recommending health standards and criteria for safety.

Under the Act, OSHA promulgates mandatory occupational safety and health standards with which employers are required to comply.

To enforce the Act, OSHA has authority to enter establishments at any time to inspect or whenever the work environment has been reported not to be in compliance with the standards; OSHA also has the authority to issue citations and assess penalties. Approximately 60 million workers in about 5 million establishments are covered by the Act in agriculture, the professions, retail and service industries, including the health care industry, as well as those in jobs generally classified as industrial(2).

IMPLICATIONS FOR NURSING

The first and most obvious implication of the Act is the mandate that it sets for those nurses who work in occupational health and are involved in activities which serve the health and safety needs of workers.

The Act assigns separate but dependent responsibilities and rights to employers and employees, and this determines the second implication. Those nurses who are employees and their employers in the health care industry have responsibilities with respect to achieving safe working conditions.

The fact that hazards in the work environment can and do cause ill health is the basis of the third implication. This mandates that information about the work environment and the patient/client's job be sought by all nurses before they make a nursing diagnosis or develop care plans.

THE OCCUPATIONAL HEALTH NURSE

Approximately 40 percent of the U.S. population work; their health is closely related to the quality of the environment in which they work. The activities of the 20,000 nurses who work in occupational health are directed in a multidisciplinary team effort toward insuring the health and safety of workers at the place of employment. Members of the occupational health team usually are a nurse, industrial hygienist, safety professional, and physician.

The nurse member frequently is the only one who works full time in an industry's occupational health unit. Success in health programs, therefore, depends upon the ability of nurses not only to work independently, but also to bring in others as needed to achieve the continued good health and safe working practices of employed persons.

The focus of the OSHA standards is environmental control. All who work in occupational health, and this includes nurses, must have an ability to detect relationships between the physical and mental ill health

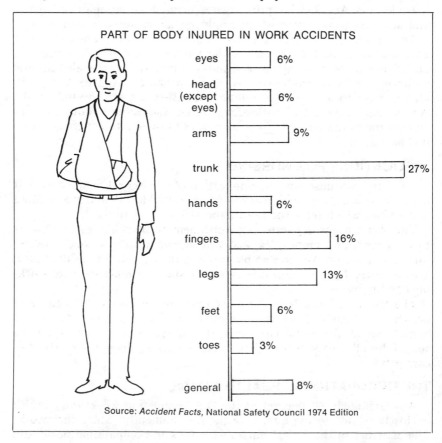

PART OF BODY INJURED IN WORK ACCIDENTS

eyes	6%
head (except eyes)	6%
arms	9%
trunk	27%
hands	6%
fingers	16%
legs	13%
feet	6%
toes	3%
general	8%

Source: *Accident Facts*, National Safety Council 1974 Edition

of workers and the stresses of their jobs. To this end, nurses make visual inspections of the processes of work and of the work areas while workers are working and assess the extent of their exposure to safety and health hazards.

Many people learned about occupational health problems, especially those associated with asbestos, when they read the articles published in the fall of 1973 in the *New Yorker* magazine(3). Although many occupational health professionals had known of the asbestos hazards, not until the Act were there federal regulations for its control.

The criteria document on asbestos prepared by NIOSH estimates that each year almost 1 million tons of asbestos are used in the United States. Inhalation of asbestos fiber produces a characteristic pattern of roentgenographic changes and physiological changes consistent with a lung disorder, such as diffuse chronic inflammation and scarring of the lung. The frequency of bronchogenic cancer, greater than expected on the basis of the general male population, was manifest among persons who worked in the manufacture of asbestos products and among those who installed asbestos insulation. Other studies showed the number of cases of mesothelioma to be excessive(4).

STANDARD FOR ASBESTOS

The first health standard promulgated by OSHA under the provision of Section 6B of PL 91-596 was for asbestos(5). This standard requires that an annual medical examination be provided for each employee exposed to five fibers of airborne asbestos longer than 5 micrometers per cubic centimeter of air. It also requires recording the symptoms of respiratory disease, chest x-ray, pulmonary function tests, and retention of the health record by the employer for at least 20 years.

STANDARD FOR VINYL CHLORIDE

The Vinyl Chloride Standard 1910.93(q) promulgated by OSHA went into effect in April 1975. This standard had its beginning on January 22, 1974, when representatives from the B. F. Goodrich Chemical Company informed NIOSH that the deaths of several employees at their Louisville, Ky., plant might have been related to occupational exposures. An immediate industrial hygiene walk-through survey of the facility was conducted by NIOSH and resulted in the agency's developing and transmitting to affected companies recommendations for precautionary monitoring and control procedures for polymerization processes involving vinyl chloride. The clustering of four cases of an unusual liver cancer within a five-year period at one plant was recognized as significant in view of the rarity of this tumor.

The vinyl chloride standard requires the employer to control the exposure "so that no worker is exposed to vinyl chloride at concentrations of greater than 1 ppm averaged over any 8-hour period." The standard also details the type of environmental monitoring and medical surveillance that must be done. Of import is the provision "that each employee shall be provided training in a program relating to the hazards of vinyl chloride and precautions for its safe use."(6).

There are more than 3 million different synthetic and natural chemicals, and industry markets 300 to 500 new chemicals each year, sometimes with less than adequate controls and little understanding of their toxic qualities. In all, some 10,000 chemicals are in industrial use in the United States. It has long been known that certain chemicals can cause cancer. The World Health Organization, for example, estimates that 85 percent of all cancer is derived from environmental sources.

Practically all occupational diseases mimic diseases found in the general population.

CHRONIC EXPOSURE

Occupation-related disease frequently has a long latency period, often 20 or more years from onset of exposure. Data which clearly distinguish the effects of massive doses intermittently received or small insults over a long period of time are not available. The same chemical may, with long-term chronic exposure, affect one organ of the body and, with high-dose exposure, affect a completely different organ. The possibility of environmental threat must be kept clearly in mind in diagnosing disease and investigating etiology. Only when this becomes standard will definitive data be available to support correction of workplace conditions.

Although some cause-effect relationships are well known—such as in lead poisoning, silicosis, and radiation sickness—others are just now becoming manifest. Examples of newly recognized occupational diseases are angiosarcoma of the liver caused by vinyl chloride and peripheral neuropathy caused by methy butyl ketone(7, 8).

All nurses, and especially occupational health nurses, must be acutely aware of man-environment health problems. They must seek information about the patient's job environment and they must look for relationships between the patients' signs and symptoms and the toxic substances and other hazards associated with the occupation.

Nurses who work in occupational health programs will be increasingly involved in education programs to meet the Act's requirement that workers have a right to know the nature of the hazards of their jobs. OSHA standards also require that employers provide medical surveillance for workers who are exposed to toxic substances. This requirement will increase the need for nurses prepared to do health assessment.

Another influence that determines an occupational health nurse's role is the fact that employees are also members of families and citizens of the community. Their workplace is a valuable community resource. The occupational health program that management provides for employees is but one facet (essentially a preventive service) of the total community health care system.

When workers are sick or injured at work, the occupational health nurse functions as a gatekeeper to the health care system and she is a provider of primary care. This responsibility is shared with the physician, just as responsibility for workers' health maintenance and for helping management make the work environment safe and in compliance with OSHA standards is shared with the safety professional and the industrial hygienist.

Occupational health nurses are finding they need to function in an ombudsman's role. They have to help workers learn their rights and use the resources available to them. Nurses must understand the Occupational Safety and Health Act and the federal agencies, OSHA and NIOSH, that it created if they are to help workers use the services established by the Act and not get lost in the bureaucratic maze.

THE COMMUNITY HEALTH NURSE

Of the 5 million establishments covered by OSHA fewer than 1 percent employ 500 or more people; hence, most establishments do not employ safety and health professionals. The Bureau of Labor Statistics estimates that only 21 percent of the workers in the private nonfarm sector had access to the services of an occupational health nurse in 1972(9).

If the other 79 percent are to have the same benefits, nurses other than those who work as occupational health nurses increasingly must be involved. The agencies for which public health nurses work must, therefore, accept what for many is a new concept: that each establishment that employs small numbers of employees and operates on a small margin of profit is, in effect, an occupational health indigent and in need of a public health service that they cannot provide for themselves.

Nurses who work out of community health agencies that accept this premise can be very effective. They can provide not only the usual public health nursing services but many of the safety and health activities the workers and management of small establishments so badly need. To be as effective in the latter as in the former, public health nurses must be knowledgeable about the Act and understand accident prevention and the etiology of occupational diseases.

Most essential is an agency administrative framework that provides nurses with access to occupational safety and health professionals when their specialized expertise is required.

Health maintenance organizations (HMOs) that have an occupational health unit, industrial clinics, and mobile health services working out of city health departments are being suggested as sources of health assessment services for workers in establishments too small to have in-plant occupational health units. Nurse practitioners with an orientation to the ecology of work, an understanding of toxicology, and knowledge of OSHA standards will be required to staff these units.

THE NURSE AS A WORKER

Hospitals are the third largest employer in the United States, with approximately 3 million employees working full and part time. Nurses are a significant part of this work force. Occupational health and safety hazards in hospitals are similar to those found in industrial and commercial establishments. In addition, there are other risks to employees unique to health care institutions.

Unfortunately, hospitals do not appear to have a consistent method for providing occupational health services for their employees nor specific criteria for such programs. General industry standards apply to the health care industry. Administrators of hospitals and nursing homes are responsible for assuring that their institutions are in compliance.

The influence that nursing service administrators and head nurses have on the management of the work areas makes it essential that they be able to identify unsafe acts and unsafe conditions, and that they not permit them to continue. For example, blocked aisles, wet floors, exit signs that are not in place, faulty electric cords, defective ladders, gas cylinders not properly stored, and blocked fire doors are dangers. They are also examples of work situations not in compliance with OSHA standards.

In a study of hospital occupational health services done by NIOSH in 1972-1973, only about half of all hospitals, regardless of size, reported having a formally organized safety and health program(10). These figures varied from 34.5 percent of the small hospitals to 70.2 percent of the large hospitals. Medium and large hospitals reported that they perform air and biological sampling in workplaces with significantly greater frequency (65.3 percent and 68.2 percent respectively) than small hospitals, 58.0 percent.

There is the same general pattern with regard to other types of environmental health and safety programs when bed size is taken into account. Survey results indicate that small hospitals—those with fewer than 100 beds—seldom have formalized environmental protective programs, while medium-sized hospitals (100 to 299 beds) tend to perform more such activities, and larger ones, generally speaking, perform still more.

Nurses as workers have rights under the Act and, because they are health professionals, they have a contribution to make to their own and to other workers' health maintenance. For example, the nurse who is pregnant and has not had measles should elect to be transferred to a less potentially dangerous area than, for example, a pediatrics unit, and all pregnant nurses should transfer from work in operating rooms.

Data collected from a retrospective study suggest that work in operating rooms carries increased risk of spontaneous abortions and congenital abnormalities in offspring, and of cancer, hepatic, and renal disease. Increase risk of congenital abnormalities also was found when the wives of men who work in the same environment were studied. The cause-effect relationship suspected is exposure to waste anesthetic gases(11).

THE NURSE AS A PROVIDER OF CARE

The patron saint of industrial medicine was Bernardino Ramazzini (1633-1714). In *The Disease of Workmen (DeMarbis Artificum Diatriba)*, he told physicians of his day to inquire without fail "of what trade are you?"(12).

The need to establish cause-and-effect relationships between work and chronic illness demands that nurses seek information about any patient's job environment.

For example, nurses who work in emergency services of hospitals need to be aware that a patient may be there because he has been overcome by chemical fumes or because he is acutely ill from exposure to a toxic substance. Others may be in the ER because they have been injured at work. It is essential that nurses ask, "Is there anything in this patient's work environment that could have contributed to his presenting condition?"

The care provided must protect workers returning to their jobs by avoiding dressings that can get caught in machinery and by not allowing patients to return to work while on drugs that decrease alertness. Effective care also includes informing employers of the suspected cause so that corrective action can be taken.

Nurses who work in specialty clinics, such as neurological, chest, dermatology, and maternity, must be particularly alert to possible occupational exposures(13). Hazards in the patient's work environment can and do cause injury to the skin(14). Such insults must be controlled if therapy is to be successful.

Nurses working in an obstetric clinic must remember that many women work, determine where each pregnant woman works, and assess the potential for harm in her environment, both to her and to the fetus(15). For example, if there is a possibility of exposure to carbon monoxide, lead, mercury, or radiation, the pregnant woman should have special protection, especially during the first trimester of the pregnancy.

The purpose of the Occupational Safety and Health Act is to preserve our human resources. Because nurses deal with so many people who are workers, nurses have a special responsibility. Every health care plan must include health and safety education so that worker/patients will learn to accept the suggested health maintenance activities and work practices that can contribute to continued health and safety(16).

THE NURSE EDUCATOR

The Occupational Safety and Health Act has important implications for those responsible for the development of curriculums for educational programs for nurse practitioners who care for adults and for occupational health nurse specialists.

Ramazzini suggested that physicians learn the nature of disease by going into the places where people work. Nurse educators will find that an assignment to an occupational health unit in industry or in hospitals permits students to learn how to provide preventive health care and health education for workers(16). Such activities provide a learning experience that permits students to interact with people who are not patients but who do need and can benefit from nursing intervention(17, 19).

SUMMARY

It has not been my intent to provide a detailed review of the implications of the Occupational Safety and Health Act of 1970 for nurses and nursing but, rather, to create an awareness of the insidious nature of many agents in the work environment that can and do cause ill health. The work environment is but one facet of the total environment, and occupational health services one part of the total health system.

Nurses as workers have the right to expect their work environment to be safe and the people to whom nurses provide care have the right to expect that nurses take into consideration the possible casual relationship of their jobs to their health problem.

The three implications selected to illustrate this article are just that: illustrations. An Act that has as its purpose "to preserve our human resources" cannot but influence those responsible for nursing education programs toward a deeper commitment to prevention and nurse practitioners to a deeper awareness that work can be hazardous to health, unless hazards in the work environment are recognized and controlled.

REFERENCES

1. OCCUPATIONAL Safety and Health Act of 1970, Public Law 91-596 (29 U.S.C. 651 et seq.)
2. U.S. PRESIDENT. *Report on Occupational Safety and Health.* (annual report for 1973) Washington, D.C., U.S. Government Printing Office, 1975.
3. BRODEUR, PAUL. Annals of industry. *New Yorker* 49:44-48ff, 92ff, 131-138ff, 87-88ff, 126ff; Oct. 26, Nov. 5, Nov. 12, Nov. 19, Nov. 26, 1973.
4. U.S. NATIONAL INSTITUTE FOR OCCUPATIONAL SAFETY AND HEALTH. *Criteria for a Recommended Standard, Occupational Exposure: to Asbestos.* (H.S.M. 72-10267) Washington, D.C., U.S. Government Printing Office, 1972.
5. ASBESTOS Standard, Title 29 Code of Federal Regulations, Section 1910.1001.
6. VINYL Chloride Standard Title 29 C.F.R., Section 1910.1017
7. CREECH, J. L., JR., AND JOHNSON, M. N. Angiosarcoma of liver in the manufacture of polyvinyl chloride. *J. Occup. Med.* 16:150-151, Mar. 1974.
8. BILIMAIRE, DONALD, AND OTHERS. Peripheral neuropathy in a coated fabrics plant. *J. Occup. Med.* 16:665-671, Oct. 1974.
9. U.S. LABOR DEPARTMENT. *Occupational Injuries and Illness by Industry, 1972.* (Bulletin No. 1830) Washington, D.C., U.S. Government Printing Office, 1974.
10. U.S. HEALTH, EDUCATION, AND WELFARE DEPARTMENT. *Hospital Occupational Health Services Study Part 1. Environmental Health and Safety Control.* (HEW Publication No. (NIOSH) 75-101) Washington, D.C., U.S. Government Printing Office, 1974.
11. AD HOC COMMITTEE. Occupational diseases among operating room personnel: a national study. *Anesthesiology* 41:321-340, Oct. 1974.
12. RAMAZZINI, BERNARDINO. *Disease of Workers;* translated from the Latin text of De Morbis Artificum by W. C. Wright. (New York Academy of Medicine Library, History of Medicine Series No. 23.) New York, Hafner Publishing Co., 1964.
13. CARNOW, B. W., AND OTHERS. A bookshelf on occupational health and safety. *Am. J. Public Health* 65:503-520, May 1975.
14. EMMITT E. A. Occupational skin cancer: a review. *J. Occup. Med.* 17:44-49, Jan. 1975.
15. U.S. WOMEN'S BUREAU. *Women Workers Today.* Washington, D.C., U.S. Government Printing Office, 1974.
16. TABERSHAW, I. R. Medical criteria for work in respiratory hazards. *J. Occup. Med.* 16:402-405, June 1974.
17. PERMANENT COMMISSION AND INTERNATIONAL ASSOCIATION ON OCCUPATIONAL HEALTH, NURSING SUBCOMMITTEE 1971-1973. *The Nurses's Contribution to the Health of the Worker—Education of the Nurse.* London, The Commission, 1974.
18. WORLD HEALTH ORGANIZATION. *Environmental and Health Monitoring in Occupational Health.* (Technical Report Series No. 535) Geneva, The Organization, 1973, p. 1.
19. U.S. PUBLIC HEALTH SERVICE, ENVIRONMENTAL HEALTH SERVICE, BUREAU OF OCCUPATIONAL SAFETY AND HEALTH. *Occupational Health Content in Baccalaureate Nursing Education,* by M. T. Keller in association with W. T. May, Cincinnati, Ohio, The Service, 1970.

From the *American Journal of Nursing* 77:433-435, Mar. 1977. Copyright © 1977. AJN Co.

Nurse-Managed Tuberculosis Clinic

LOIS D. PETERSON • JUANITA H. GREEN

With personal attention and individualized nursing care, "unreliable" tuberculosis patients became regulars at a nurse-managed clinic.

"I don't give a damn about your excuses, you just get yourself over here PRONTO and get your shot."

This blunt telephone advice from one patient attending our nurse-managed clinic to another illustrates the camaraderie among patients who previously were considered irresponsible about their health care.

The clinic had been functioning for about two years and, we believed, functioning successfully. To verify our impression, we traced what had happened to the patients admitted between June 1972, when the clinic opened, through October 1974.

In the early 1970s, the Miami Veterans Administration Hospital was following the national trend of early discharge for tuberculosis patients, with referral to its pulmonary clinic. However, the clinic population had grown too large for the available physicians to manage adequately, some patients were unable to follow the recommended self-care regimen, many failed to take their prescribed medications, and some did not return for regular follow-up.

LOIS D. PETERSON, R.N., B.S.N., *is the discharge planning public health nurse co-ordinator, Miami Veterans Administration Hospital, Fla.* JUANITA H. GREEN, R.N., M.P.H., *is the nursing supervisor of ambulatory care, Miami Veterans Administration Hospital. The authors appreciate the support of George Baum, M.D., associate professor of medicine, University of Miami School of Medicine, and Arthur Schwartz, M.D., staff physician, ambulatory care medicine clinics, Miami Veterans Administration Hospital, and thank Gracie Wyche, R.N., and Nereida Lawrence, R.N., who staffed the nurse-managed clinic.*

Evaluating Candidates for Nurse-Clinic

2—has home with "interested other"
2—is not an alcoholic
1—does not smoke or stopped when instructed to
1—first tuberculosis treatment period
1—employed or has regular income
1—has history of successful self-care in another
    condition requiring medication
1—receptive toward regimen
1—responds to and is interested in health education

10—highest possible score

Inpatients scoring less than 5 are considered for intermittent therapy

So, with great interest and support from the nursing and medical staff, we started a nurse-managed tuberculosis intermittent therapy clinic for those patients who, we hoped, would respond to extra instruction and extra attention from the nursing staff.

Our goals were to prevent rehospitalization, to keep the patients noninfectious, and to retain them in treatment as long as medically indicated. The nurses primarily involved in the clinic were the public health nurse coordinator, the charge nurse of the tuberculosis outpatient clinic, and the outpatient clinic nursing supervisor.

The public health nurse coordinator and a social service worker used an informally devised reliability scale, ranking patients from 0 to 10 when making recommendations for the nurse-clinic. Patients who ranked below five on the scale were considered for the nurse-clinic.

Final decision for referral rested with our interdisciplinary discharge planning group, composed of physicians, a social worker, the head nurse of the inpatient unit, and the public health nursing coordinator.

INPATIENT CARE

The public health nurse coordinator talked with patients as soon as possible after their admission to the hospital. She began teaching them about tuberculosis and obtained information for the health department's communicable disease report. Discussing this report with the patient provided an opportunity to talk about infectiousness, methods of control, the need for prolonged treatment, and the need to protect others.

A social worker also saw the patient, early, to identify family problems, financial difficulties, and other problems created by hospitalization. The interdisciplinary discharge planning group attempted early identification of patients who might benefit from intermittent therapy.

A patient group met weekly. The physician, staff nurses, social service personnel and public health nurse coordinator presented formal material. The physician discussed lung physiology, showing the patients their x-rays that demonstrated active tuberculosis, and emphasizing the success of consistent and prolonged treatment.

The nurses discussed ways to prevent the spread of organisms and the kinds of medications and side effects, and reinforced the need for long treatment. Laboratory personnel described culture techniques, illustrating them with cultures positive for acid-fast bacilli. Free discussion was encouraged, and a social worker assisted. Representatives of the local health department and lung association participated in several classes.

Weekly interdisciplinary ward rounds included the nurse from the outpatient clinic. During this time the patient was informed of his progress and the plans for his discharge. When the interdisciplinary team decided that a patient was ready for discharge to the nurse-clinic, the public health nurse coordinator took him on a tour of the entire outpatient clinic and introduced the nurses who would be responsible for his follow-up care.

NURSE-CLINIC CARE

The public health nurse coordinator sent a registry card to the outpatient clinic with the physician's orders for intermittent therapy. The patient received a card with the date of his first appointment, room number, and names and phone numbers of at least two nurses to call if he had any questions.

Between June 1972 and October 1974, we followed 15 patients who had been hospitalized for an average of 61 days. At discharge from the hospital, 13 of them had negative sputum specimens; two had positive specimens.

Our patients, who attended the nurse-managed clinic twice a week for an average of six-and-a-half months, attended the physician clinic once a month. Appointments were arranged around the patients' work schedules, and patients were expected to call the clinic nurse if an appointment could not be kept or if they developed side effects from their medications.

One or the other of two clinic nurses ran the clinic sessions. The nurse assumed full control of the nurse-managed clinic and employed public health nursing skills. She completed an initial assessment of all patients and monitored vital signs and weight weekly.

All antituberculosis medications were given by the nurses during the clinic sessions. These usually included combinations of streptomycin sulfate and isoniazid (INH) or ethambutal hydrochloride and INH. Pyridoxine hydrochloride (vitamin B_6) was given to prevent peripheral neuritis caused by isoniazid. The nurse reviewed the possible side effects from these medications.

On a monthly basis, the nurse referred patients to the physician clinic and obtained sputum smears and cultures. She collaborated with the physician in the pulmonary clinic if problems occurred. When indicated, she referred patients to other departments, such as social service or dietary.

The nurse attended chest conference and tuberculosis rounds weekly. She kept the tuberculosis registry up-to-date, recorded pertinent information, and telephoned or wrote patients when necessary. For example, a patient whose sputum became positive would be scheduled to see the physician and all patients who failed to attend a clinic session were contacted.

Two thirds of the patients completed the prescribed regimen in the nurse-clinic and only one was lost to follow-up.

We believe there are several reasons for the clinic's success:

Patient Attitudes. The respect and enthusiasm of the staff seemed to enable each patient to grow a little in responsibility to himself and to other patients. As the program progressed, fewer patients arrived at the clinic intoxicated, and those who did were usually apologetic.

As patients learned more about tuberculosis, they became less fearful of the disease and more hopeful about recovery. They showed continued interest in their progress and responded to the reinforcement of instruction.

Continuity of Staff. The two clinic nurses came to know all the patients well. This was one clear advantage over the regular pulmonary clinic. Having "my nurse" became highly important, reflecting a kind of trust that is not easily established.

Patient Education. Just the act of instructing, whether individually or in groups, said to these patients: "We think you are worthy. We believe you can learn. We need your help in achieving your recovery."

Nurse-Managed Intermittent Therapy
June 1972 to October 1974

Profile of 15 patients: age range, 34-66 yrs; average age, 51.5

Extent of disease
    Far advanced   11
    Moderately advanced   3
    Minimally advanced   1

Hospitalization(s) for tuberculosis
    One   10
    Two   3
    Three   1
    Four   1

Personal/social
    History of successfully taking medication
      for another condition   3
    Admitted to heavy drinking   10
    Admitted to heavy smoking   13
    Lived alone   7
    Lived with immediate family or with "interested other"   8
    Long history of unemployment   6
    Worked occasionally   4
    Worked full time   5
    Response to ward routine and inpatient teaching
      Good   9
      Fair   5
      Poor   1

Results of 15 Patients' Intermittent Therapy

Completed prescribed regimen in clinic
  and transferred to regular follow-up   11
Lost to follow-up   1
Died from condition unrelated to tuberculosis   1
Continued to attend clinic   2
Rehospitalized for tuberculosis   0
Positive sputum specimens occurring
  after discharge from hospital   0

Attendance at the intermittent therapy clinic continues to be regular. We believe that our methods can work in other situations with other kinds of patients.

Staff Attitudes. All staff members wanted the program to succeed and their enthusiasm "infected" patients. Their total acceptance of the patient and his life-style appeared to have positive effects on his behavior. The staff acted on the premise that "uninformed does not mean unintelligent," and this created a comfortable atmosphere for everyone.

The patient was welcomed at the clinic even if he arrived drunk and unkempt, and he was praised for his effort in keeping the appointment. He was not kept waiting, even though he might arrive much later than his scheduled appointment. Several patients commented that they had seldom been treated this way.

An indication of the clinic's success was the expansion of the nurse-clinic. In addition to the intermittent therapy clinic, the nurses now conduct clinic sessions for all tuberculosis outpatients. All patients discharged from the hospital return once to the physician clinic, and then attend a nurse-managed tuberculosis clinic for their second and third visits. A fourth visit is scheduled in the physician clinic. Between physician visits, our clinic nurses monitor the patients' progress as in the intermittent therapy clinic. They also perform vision tests on all patients to detect side effects of ethambutal hydrochloride, and order chest x-rays and blood work (CBC, SGOT, SGPT).

Success of any nurse-managed clinic, we believe, depends on nurse enthusiasm, physician and social service support, early contact with hospitalized patients, personal attention to the patient in transition from hospital to home, and continuous reinforcement of all measures to maintain health.

From the *American Journal of Nursing* 76:592-593, Apr. 1976. Copyright © 1976. AJN Co.

A College Contraceptive Clinic

SUSAN W. ANDREWS

Unwanted pregnancies and venereal diseases have decreased at this small New Hampshire college since a clinic was opened at which counseling is stressed and prescriptions and referrals are provided.

"Why can't I go on and off the pill whenever I need to? My boyfriend goes to another college, and we see each other only a few times during the school year." "My periods are irregular. Will I ever become pregnant?" "What does a diaphragm do?" These and other sex-related questions are asked every day of college health nurses all over the country.

At New England College, Henniker, New Hampshire, we have developed a contraceptive program which many of the 1,200 students use.

Since the contraceptive program was started in 1972, sex-related problems have decreased on campus. At the close of the second year of the program, requests for diagnostic tests for pregnancy had dropped 50 percent, and the percentage of positive tests for pregnancy had dropped 26 percent. Also, venereal disease reports were down 24 percent.

More students than ever are using our services. Approximately 22 percent of the total female population were seen in our program during the first year and last year 34 percent were seen. Our screening tests have uncovered cases of gonorrhea that might otherwise have gone undetected for a dangerously long time.

Unfortunately, our clinic has not attracted many men students, although 65 percent of the student population are men. We are planning a public relations campaign to bring more men into the program. Couples come in for contraceptive and VD counseling.

SUSAN ANDREWS, R.N., *is a staff nurse in the New England College Health Center, Henniker, N. H.*

Clinic use does not tell the whole story. We find students we talk with are better informed and students are coming to the health center increasingly with other health problems.

Before a woman can make an appointment with the clinic, she must attend an informal contraception information session, which a nurse leads one evening weekly. Individual sessions are arranged if the student does not feel comfortable in a group. Sessions are mandatory for two reasons.

First, the information we wish to convey (anatomy and physiology of the male and female reproductive systems, hygiene, methods of birth control, venereal diseases, self breast examination, and vaginal examination) is given in systematic and organized fashion, with a general discussion and question-and-answer period following. Second, it saves time.

We use the excellent film, *Hope Is Not a Method*[1] to cover the subject of methods. We offer additional information on venereal diseases and menstrual extraction.

We do not recommend one contraceptive method over another, but present the facts objectively and let the student decide. It is amazing how much misinformation students reveal. For example, one girl was convinced that her "safe" time of the month was mid-menstrual cycle. Many students have only vague knowledge regarding reproductive anatomy in both sexes.

At this group session, appointments are arranged for the girls who wish to take the pill. They write information about their family and personal histories, which is kept on file at the health center. When they come for their appointment, the doctor reviews it. When necessary, further individual counseling is arranged.

As for the time saving, the girls still ask questions when they come to the health center for individual appointments, but not nearly as many as they did before. When there is a tight schedule, saving time is important.

Women who wish to use a diaphragm or intrauterine device are referred to gynecologists in nearby Concord. We make appointments for them and they are seen promptly. Women who wish to use the pill are seen by our health center physician or college health nurse practitioner.

The remaining birth control methods are withdrawal, rhythm, chemical methods, and condoms. Students seldom choose withdrawal and rhythm, but we counsel students who desire to use them. We urge an appointment with a gynecologist.

---

[1]The film is available through Perennial Education, Inc., 1825 Willow Rd., Northfield, Ill. 60093. Color, Running time, 16 minutes. Purchase price, $200. Rental, $20. It is suitable for junior and senior high-school students and college students.

Foams and condoms are for sale at cost through the health center and the head residents in the dormitories. When necessary, appropriate instructions and cautions are given at the time of purchase. As far as the sale of condoms goes, men outnumber women in buying them, but last year we noticed more and more women coming in for them.

Women new to the pill have follow-up visits every three months for the first year to assess their physical progress, and we are available to answer questions that may arise or give reassurance when necessary. If any untoward symptoms are evident, we refer students to the doctor. After the first year, the girls return only every six months.

Our patients are required to have a vaginal examination, breast examination, and repeat screening tests once a year. Screening tests include a Pap smear for cytologic classification, cellular analysis, and estrogen effect, cervical and anal smears for gonorrhea (transgrow medium and methylene blue); and a monilial culture on Nickerson's medium. If indicated, we test for such vaginal infections as trichomonas. Students are encouraged to return any time problems arise.

Pregnancy tests are handled throughout the year, and the nurse reports the test results to the girl. When it is positive, some girls react hysterically. We sound the girl out gently and tell her that perhaps the best time to discuss her options will be later, when she is in better control of herself. This works well and gives the student a breather from the shock.

The majority of pregnant students opt for abortion. In three years, I know of only one girl who decided to continue her pregnancy to term. The student decides where she will have the abortion. Some go home. Some go out of state. Most go to a local hospital or women's services center.

Follow-up counseling is provided to encourage the student to adopt a birth control method and to help her vent her feelings after the abortion. Counseling can be continued for as long as necessary.

One unfortunate young woman became pregnant after a single sexual contact. She also contracted gonorrhea, had a late D and C, and ended up with monilial and then trichomonas infections. Needless to say, she required counseling for a long time.

If the woman decides to bear her child, necessary aid can be obtained from such outside resources as the "Right to Life" organizations.

With venereal diseases so wide-spread, one inevitably encounters cases on the college campus. As with pregnancy, venereal disease counseling is handled throughout the year. Slides and smears are processed at the health center. VDRL are sent to the state laboratory in Concord, where service is free. The laboratory reports are returned within 10 days.

We stress confidentiality when a student has VD, as we do with all aspects of the contraceptive control program. We hope that we are conveying no stigma of moral judgment, which will enable students to use our services without shame or embarrassment.

For such vaginal infections as monilia and trichomonas, standing orders allow the nurse to institute treatment after appropriate testing. We encourage the girls to return for follow-up testing after treatment. If the girl has a steady sexual partner, he also may require treatment.

We provide a wide variety of pills at no cost to the students. New Hampshire law makes charging for medication illegal except for pharmacies.

Condoms and foam were at first free. They are now sold at cost. Foam prices vary, but a reliable brand of condoms sells for $1.00 a dozen.

When a woman requests an IUD or diaphragm, we make the appointment, but she must meet the expense. Fortunately, there are women's clinics in Concord which provide the services of gynecologists on the basis of ability to pay. This is less expensive than the $25 cost for private patients. Very recently, our nurse practitioner learned to fit diaphragms. We added this service to our clinic and charge the student for the diaphragm and lubricant only. If she prefers a gynecologist, we set up the appointment for her.

The health center absorbs other costs, including lab tests, the college physician's services, medications in stock, and teaching literature.

Opportunities to learn new skills at workshops, such as learning to do pelvics, are seized eagerly by the nurses. Our school physician follows up these learning experiences with guidance and observation.

We nurses have to be sure that our knowledge of contraception is current. Some of the students are sharp on the subject. Recently, one 20-year-old woman helped me out during a counseling session by correctly explaining how the FSH and LH hormones affect the menstrual cycle.

Another student brightened my evening not long ago by exclaiming, "You're great! I didn't know there was someone like you to talk to."

From the *American Journal of Nursing* 76:274-275, Feb. 1976. Copyright © 1976. AJN Co.

Rural Mobile Health Unit

VIRGINIA L. BARKER

A clinic on wheels is giving access to health care to residents of a thinly populated area in New York State.

The old picture: a physician, in a horse-drawn buggy, making patient rounds down country lanes.

New picture: the mobile health unit, a nurse-staffed, 35-foot vehicle touring the country roads of Allegany County, N. Y.

The unit serves an area of 75,000 square miles with a population, according to the 1970 U. S. Census, of 45,458. There are no cities in the area, only small villages or clusters of houses, and 15 percent of the population is over 60 years of age, with many of the residents having incomes well below the poverty level.

These days there are only 18 primary care physicians in the county. The majority of these are over 65, several in their late 70s; most are general practitioners. The isolation of the area has made it difficult for the doctors to get away for postgraduate study, and their care is illness oriented.

The Alfred University School of Nursing and Health Care Mobile Health Unit went on the road in 1972, under a grant from the Lakes Area Regional Medical Program, as a project of the Alfred University School of Nursing and Health Care. Now the university has taken over the financing.

Where the physician in the horse-drawn buggy focused on illness, the unit's focus is on health. The vehicle is completely self-contained, with power generator, water supply, and toilet. The interior is divided into a

VIRGINIA BARKER, R.N., Ed.D., *is dean of the Alfred University College of Nursing and Health Care, Alfred, New York.*

reception area and two examining rooms, plus a miniscule half bath and a combination audiometric testing chamber/dressing room.

The staff at any one site consists of two nurses from the Allegany County Public Health Nursing Service and the driver-secretary. The nurses change with the different locations; they serve on the unit when it is scheduled in their district. During the academic year, sophomore and senior Alfred nursing students receive part of their clinical experience in community health nursing on the unit.

The unit makes monthly visits to seven sites in the county, with the precise location of the sites changing as the need varies. The schedule is publicized by radio, newspaper, service clubs, churches, school groups, and the like. Services are free to the public and include health education classes and health assessment examinations of children under six years and adults 18 years and over. (The ages between are covered by the school health services.) The educational programs are carried out in churches and community centers.

One major benefit derived from the unit is the early identification of health problems. A patient with problems is counseled by the public health nurses and referred to his or her family physician. A letter is sent to the doctor explaining that the person has visited the unit and the reason for the referral. If the person has no physician, the nurses provide a list from which to make a choice. Some time later—the time depending on the severity of the problem—a nurse follows up. If the client has seen a doctor, she helps him carry out the physician's orders. If the client has not made an appointment, the nurse tries to determine the reason—lack of transportation or funds or whatever—and then tries to solve the problem.

We know we are meeting residents' need for some kind of entry into the health care system. A survey of our clients revealed that the average length of time since they were seen by a doctor was 10 years. Recently, we saw one who had not seen a physician professionally for 40 years. Initially, it was anticipated that the referral rate would be around 40 percent. In actuality, the referral rate for adults is 90 percent and for children 34 percent. We are finding, too, that a client is likely to need to be referred for more than one health problem.

Our immediate plans call for the addition of more health education classes—classes for diabetics, classes in child growth and development, and classes in economical nutrition for all ages. We plan also to determine whether, as a result of the mobile health unit's activity, area residents' health related activities change in a way that indicates a change in regard to health care from illness to health orientation.

Physician support is growing slowly. We had been concerned lest we overwhelm the available doctors with referrals, but this has not happened. We believe the health counseling and the early case-finding activities will assist the doctors by freeing them to devote their energies to individuals needing curative medical care.

From *MCN The American Journal of Maternal Child Nursing* 1:88-92, Mar.-Apr. 1976. Copyright © 1976. AJN Co.

Camp Nursing: An Opportunity for Independent Practice in a Miniature Community

HOLLIS A. BACKMAN ● **NANCY J. PACKARD** ● **ANN C. REINER**

Camping can be an opportunity for a nurse at any level, not only a new graduate, to exercise the expanded roles of health care delivery. These nurses give an example of how this can be done.

Despite the persistence of limited perceptions of what camp nurses do, summer camp can be an occasion for nurses to experiment in the expanded capacities of planning, coordinating, and providing comprehensive health care for a small and insular community. If the nurse tries out these roles as well as the one of providing conventional services such as emergency first aid, changing dressings, dispensing personal medications, and reassuring homesick campers, camp will not be merely a fun or easy place in which to work. It will challenge the individual's mental energy, improvisational skills, and physical stamina as we found our camp did.

Although each nurse's experience will be as singular as the camp involved, those nurses who have identified the potential for autonomy in nursing can realize that autonomy in the independent camp nursing role. We did so through the planner/coordinator/provider model.

The first level, nurse as planner, implies a beginning; at this stage we developed our camp health center philosophies and set up short- and long-term goals for ourselves as individual practitioners and as a nursing team. Our objectives were threefold: Because our population was relatively healthy upon arrival, we wanted to help campers and staff to become aware and heedful of their physical and emotional well-being, and in so doing, to prevent illness by maintaining health.

We would seek to encourage in campers and staff members a sense of personal responsibility for their own health care—responsibility which includes the dimensions of patient involvement in decision making and active participation in the plan of care. Finally, we would try to provide care that suited the needs of the whole person and not merely those resulting from an isolated incident.

Our attempts to promote health and assist in its maintenance were most successful when the individuals involved understood the concepts behind our care. Accordingly, patient teaching was our predominant technique in promoting health.

Our health care instruction began with a detailed first-aid session for the staff during training week. Later we held workshops with the campers covering basic first aid and hygiene for canoeing, backpacking, and extended sailing trips, which were the focus of camp activities. Specific areas covered with the campers were the necessary supplies in a first-aid kit and first-aid techniques, with major emphasis on needs that arise on the trail such as care of cuts, scratches, blisters, burns, and sprains.

We also explored preventive safety measures such as keeping feet covered when walking around campsites and while swimming in unknown waters; proper cleaning of dishes; care of feet while backpacking; and precautions against sunburn, heat exhaustion, and heat stroke when sailing. Because of our firm belief in the need for the individual to be responsible for and actively involved in his or her own health care and because these campers were old enough to understand the implications of such a responsibility, we also tried to teach principles such as those of good hygiene and diet and related procedures which they could take home and use.

COUNSELORS' ROLE IN HEALTH TEACHING

To assist them in their health-teaching role, we invited counselors to use our textbooks for further reference on first aid as well as for finding out about campers' medical problems. Before the beginning of a new

MS. BACKMAN, R.N., *is a staff nurse in neurology at University Hospital South in Portland, Oregon.* MS. PACKARD, R.N., *is a nurse practitioner in surgery and orthopedics at the University of Washington Hospital.* MS. REINER, R.N., *is currently a graduate student in psychosocial nursing at the University of Washington. The three nurses worked together in a camp after their graduation from St. Olaf College Department of Nursing in the summer of 1975. This article is based on their joint experience.*

camping session, we also distributed lists alerting counselors to specific camper health concerns, and they frequently consulted us about such common problems as asthma, hyperactivity, allergies, or physical limitations.

The counselors' increased awareness of health needs not only made them better teachers and models for the campers, but prompted them to provide us with the feedback necessary for proper follow-up care. Thus, the position of the counselor as a vital link in total camp health care was reaffirmed.

Patient teaching wore a more informal guise when we acted as facilitators during "interest sessions." These forum-like gatherings, held at least once during each camp session, emphasized flexibility of subject matter, and topics ranged from anatomy and physiology to sex and male/female roles in society. Anyone who was interested could come, and we overcame participants' hesitancy to ask questions or express concerns by allowing them to submit their questions anonymously on scraps of paper which were "drawn from a hat" and read aloud. This method stimulated thought and provoked responses from even the most reticent individuals.

As another method of communicating health knowledge, we made literature available to the campers. We did this in a very casual manner, leaving it on tables in the health center waiting room. Most of the material consisted of pamphlets and booklets written for the general public and offered by various health promotion organizations. We tried to choose those most appropriate to the adolescent and the situation at hand. Among the subjects examined in them were nutrition, venereal disease, safety on the trail, the dangers of smoking, and birth control. We also provided, for staff and campers, literature on the concept of the "well body" and the sociomedical trend toward viewing the patient as a consumer of health care.

Maintaining good health was especially important in our setting since the activities of camp life demanded that those enrolled be in good physical condition. Similarly, staff members had to stay well in order to work the long hours required and to remain consistently attentive to the ever-changing needs of the individual campers. Camp regulations and procedures therefore ensured sufficient periods for rest and sleep and availability of adequate food and emphasized proper body mechanics and using tools safely.

Periodic health checkups, carried out at least three times during each camp session, were also significant in the program of health maintenance. Upon their arrival, campers were given abbreviated physical exams by volunteer doctors, who reviewed health history forms for incomplete areas and recommended treatments pertinent to specific health concerns. During this check-in procedure, we introduced ourselves and the health center facilities to the campers and collected personal medications, noted the status of everyone's tetanus booster, and collaborated with the physicians on care plans.

During the course of the campers' stay, they were also required to pass through the health center before leaving for the trail and immediately upon returning. At these times we packed their personal medications and instructions for use in their first-aid kits, took each one's temperature, and verbally checked for any complaints, particularly of upper respiratory infections. We also took the opportunity to inspect for athlete's foot and apply antifungal medications when necessary.

This was an important part of our care, for camp life provided the ideal environment for growth of athlete's foot fungus. To save equipment from unnecessary damage "wet foot" canoeing was practiced. That is, campers waded into the water to load and board the canoe instead of doing so on shore. What's more, instead of allowing the canoe to ram into shore when they arrived at their destination, one of the campers was expected to get out and gently pull it to shore. As a result, the campers and counselors often went through the day with wet feet, having an opportunity to dry their feet and boots only after their campsite has been set up for the night.

A regimen of self-care in foot hygiene was continually encouraged to stave off this problem and also to prevent incapacitating blisters and infections in backpackers, who were very prone to them. Campers soon learned that they could not neglect their feet or they would have to pay the consequences of being unable to participate in activities.

We conducted the last health check at the end of each session, when we recorded for later evaluation differences in health status in each of the campers from the time he or she had entered three weeks earlier. We gave simple instructions to campers for continuing at home any treatments we had started and wrote letters to parents when more involved care or follow-up by local physicians was needed. Then we returned medications that the campers had brought along and again offered our help as resource persons during the inevitable going-home confusion.

Although we used numerous and often variable approaches to meeting our goal of maintaining health, this only reflected our emphasis on caring for the whole, individual person. The degree to which a person assumed responsibility in the care plan helped illustrate the viability of our campaign. Whether it was a tired staff member who came to the health center for rest and privacy or a camper who "just wanted to talk," we were encouraged when people were aware enough of their needs to respond to them while prevention of illness was still possible. At such times we felt we had filled the first role outlined by the planner/coordinator/provider model.

NURSE AS COORDINATOR

As health care coordinators, we turned to the multidisciplinary quality of community health nursing to lend us theories we could apply to our work in the camp community. Because people closely and constantly worked, played, and lived together, harmony and efficiency depended on an open exchange of ideas. And fortunately collaboration among the different factions of camp was a given factor and served us well in our efforts as facilitators.

We also relied on this spirit of cooperation in coordinating health care: we expected our fellow staff members to take an active part in community health matters and so described to them what we believed were our responsibilities to them as well as our specific expectations of them. They responded in kind. We found we could trust counselors to provide us with information about their campers' health, just as we could depend on the educated kitchen staff's use of principles of sanitation and nutrition in their food preparation.

Ideally, those who would be affected by a decision were involved in making it. For example, when a camper due to leave on a trip was in the beginning stage of a cold, we did not arbitrarily decide that he or she must remain in camp. Rather, we discussed with the camper and counselor what would be involved in going (or staying). What would be the physical demands of the trip? Could the individual successfully meet those demands? What provisions could be made to bring the person back to camp should his or her condition become worse? Although ultimately it was the nurse who had to determine what action would be most appropriate, camper, counselor, and nurse together would try to reach a decision which would satisfy all concerned.

Coordinating this process was sometimes a complicated affair, particularly when decisions were not unanimous. But attempting to include campers in decisions about their own health care was gratifying to us when it became apparent that they wanted to be a determining force and were willing to accept the outcome of decisions they had helped to reach.

NURSE AS PROVIDER

In the context of provider, we discovered we were performing many traditional nursing functions. In the health center, open 24 hours a day, crisis care occupied the largest share of time that we spent with our clients. Emergency first aid was a typical mode of intervention, and the cases we treated ranged in severity from minor burns and sprains to eye injuries and lacerations requiring further attention.

We made medical judgments in accordance with standing orders issued by the camp medical committee, which allowed us to dispense prescription medications for such conditions as external otitis, conjunctivitis, allergic reactions, and certain upper respiratory infections based on our assessment of the person. Referrals for medical attention were made in situations requiring procedures we did not perform, for example, suturing, taking x-rays for suspected fractures, and lab work.

Campers who wanted to participate actively in their own care were encouraged to do so. Under our supervision, they cleansed and dressed minor abrasions, prepared their own foot-soak solutions, and were responsible for applying unsterile hot packs. In addition to increasing patient involvement in care, these practices help our health education efforts, putting to good use the concept that one of the best ways to learn is to do.

A part of providing comprehensive nursing care for the residents of a camp community includes caring for inpatients. The transition from outpatient to inpatient status occurred when we saw the need for a person to remain in the health center for increased rest, closer observation, or isolation. Seldom did the length of stay exceed two days. For a patient whose condition demanded more intricate nursing care, we developed a written plan which could be implemented using primary nursing. Our charting was based on the problem-oriented method of recording; and we found this kept the information readily available for use after the person returned to his or her cabin.

Since we wanted to offer our clients care as free from interruption as possible, we consulted camper health history forms and charting from previous years, hoping to identify patterns of illness, and in doing so, to prevent or at least minimize those factors which might contribute to recurrence of past problems. This preventive aspiration was not always met due to various limitations such as lack of consistency in camper histories and a shortage of adequate time, but it did show some results. For example, if in reviewing a camper's history we discovered an individual's susceptibility to upper respiratory infections, by informing the counselor of this proneness we might prevent or at least detect early in its course such a problem. The counselor was thus a key contributor to prevention.

Primary nursing's appeal to us stemmed from our belief that it was a good way to deliver unfragmented care. Accordingly, we believed that follow-up was crucial. Pursuing the outcome of a camper's treatment was not difficult when the person was still in camp—we could make inquiries and suggestions during mealtimes when everyone in camp was gathered in one place. But once a camper went home, this became more difficult. We had to write and phone local physicians and parents, explaining what had been and what remained to be done.

It was important to us as providers that we remain flexible in our approach and methods of problem solving. There were outside considerations which filtered into our philosophies of care: we complied with standards set by the Wisconsin Nurse Practice Act, and we followed guidelines given us by the American Camping Association. And, of course, there were our own limitations, which could not help touching our delivery of care. Besides the element of not having enough time, we confronted fluctuating personal energy levels and a caseload which seemed overwhelming in moments when we were fatigued or ill. We had to take all of this into account during problem solving, and we tried to keep alternatives fresh in our minds—alternatives we could extract and use when existing approaches grew stale and unworkable.

A REALISTIC, INSULAR MODEL

Without the presence of institutional surroundings, the camp setting was very much like an experimental design. Few outside influences intruded into the isolated community; it was free from such intervening variables as institutional hierarchy and red tape. How fortunate we were to be in this environment among supportive people. How pleasantly accidental was our discovery that because of its insulated quality, the camp was not necessarily an unrealistic place, but could offer insights which might be applied to a larger, multifaceted community.

Camp nursing was more to us than a fun-filled summertime diversion —it was a satisfying avenue for experiencing independent practice. Through it we had the opportunity to actualize many of our professional and personal goals, and if we can retain the focus of care we acquired in that uncluttered setting, we should be able to enlarge on it and carry it with us throughout our professional careers.

For those nurses who seek greater autonomy in their practice, the traditional summer camp experience could become a seedbed for professional growth. Opportunities providing such an experience are widespread. It will be through professional incentive and creativity that our growth will become a reality.

From the *American Journal of Nursing* 75:1137-1139, July 1975. Copyright © 1975. AJN Co.

Nursing by Telephone

DONNA MURPHY • ELEANOR DINEEN

How nurses ease the care problems for the 36,000 subscribers in a health maintenance organization, where 50 percent of the visits are made by phone.

The telephone is not generally considered to be a primary tool in the delivery of nursing care. But at the Harvard Community Health Plan, it is fast becoming just that.

The Harvard Community Health Plan is a health maintenance organization serving 36,000 members in Boston and the surrounding area. The plan emphasizes preventive care and provides complete ambulatory health care services at two main health centers, a satellite center, in patients' homes when necessary, and through telephone consultation. Today, many nurses provide primary health care over the phone.

This role has evolved during the past six years since the plan was established. During the early years, so many telephone calls came in daily concerning enrollment that the staff couldn't handle them and care for patients. So a full-time position of tele-nurse was established.

A nurse, handicapped by arthritis, was recruited for the job since she had the necessary skill and knowledge for the work. Originally this nurse answered all calls herself, moving from desk to desk as the phone rang. Her records for a time consisted of pink telephone slips. Later, she added the physicians' schedule, a communicable disease book, *The Merck Manual,* a medication reference, and the poison control center number.

The need for a quiet, controlled environment eventually took her into

DONNA MURPHY, R.N., B.S., *was until recently a triage nurse in the Harvard Community Health Plan, Boston, Mass.* ELEANOR DINEEN, R.N., B.S., *is educational coordinator in the Harvard Community Health Plan and was the full-time tele-nurse there.*

her own office and a telephone head set relieved her neck strain and allowed her to keep both hands free for writing, using reference material, and so forth. The tele-nurse was eventually attached administratively to the triage service, which provides care to adult members who have not yet had their initial health visit and whose health problems require care within 24 to 48 hours.

After a time, the tele-nurse became overburdened and an expeditor was hired. She answered incoming calls and did the initial screening in the primary care areas. The expeditor referred patients to the correct person or department, obtained laboratory results and records when needed, and arranged for the patient to be called back. The expeditor recorded the name, birthdate, primary doctor, telephone number, and immediate problem.

This freed the tele-nurse to give undivided attention to each patient problem and relieved her of much paper work. If the call was an emergency, the tele-nurse responded immediately. If not, she returned the calls as the nursing work-load allowed. As her role evolved, other nurses—usually to the extent each was comfortable—began to use the telephone in the way she used it. She is now formalizing the telephone role for other nurses.

We no longer have one full-time tele-nurse. Since maximum enrollment has been achieved, calls of this type are down. Instead, use of the telephone is being incorporated into ongoing patient care and nurses in each area have their own call hours and handle their own patients during regular working hours. Expeditors continue in their initial screening role. In internal medicine, each nurse has call hours twice a day. Patients are encouraged to telephone to speak directly with the nurse. Each nurse handles approximately 5 to 20 calls per session.

In OB-GYN, one nurse is assigned as telephone coverage nurse to handle incoming calls and walk-in patients every day, and she averages 25 patients. In pediatrics, each primary team devotes one-half hour in each session to telephone calls and walk-ins; the department averages 80 to 100 calls. The nurses in the triage area share an average of 30 to 50 calls per day. A recent telephone survey in the health center revealed that 50 percent of patient care was given by telephone.

HANDLING PATIENT PROBLEMS

Nurses can circumvent the busy central appointment desk and arrange for a physician appointment, call a patient into the triage (emergency) area for immediate evaluation, or offer symptomatic treatment and send out prescriptions with physician liaison.

Patients who do require a doctor or nurse visit, for instance those with a possible fracture or urinary tract infection, can have their visit expedited. Nurses send patients to x-ray or the laboratory before they visit in the specific clinical unit.

Sally E., who lives 30 miles away, reports she severely lacerated her thumb. She is told to go to the nearest emergency department, while Robert W. from downtown Boston can take two aspirin, finish his dinner and take a subway to a six o'clock appointment for a throat culture. Guided by established standing orders, nurses often carry patients through an illness or a crisis.

The telephone interview, intended to determine when a patient should be seen, reveals a vivid clinical picture: "What is your temperature? When did your symptoms start? Are you coughing? What are you coughing up? Does your chest hurt at all?"

The guidelines in the standing orders include a list of specific symptoms to elicit from the patient in each disease category and indicate when a patient should be called in or referred to a physician. For example, an uncomplicated low-back pain—"It just started when I bent. No, the pain doesn't shoot anywhere. I'm not allergic to any medicine,"— does not necessitate a painful, possibly injurious trip to the health center. The home situation is reviewed, the patient is advised on bedrest and other treatment, and daily telephone contact is scheduled to follow the patient's progress.

EVENINGS AND WEEKENDS

Triage nurses staff the phones after regular working hours from 5:00 to 9:00 P.M., on Saturdays from 8:30 A.M. to 8:00 P.M., on Sundays and holidays from 8:30 A.M. to 6:00 P.M. These nurses also see and evaluate patients who come in. Their telephone role differs in that calls must necessarily be shorter and are geared toward treating immediate problems or referring the patient to the correct daytime person. Nurses who provide coverage evenings and weekends continue to manage new fevers, send patients with fractures to emergency wards, and calm hysterical patients.

Triage nurses process calls to all departments and refer to the physician on call those matters that they cannot handle according to standing orders. The heaviest after-hours load is for adult patients in medicine and pediatrics. On weekends and holidays the triage nurses arrange patient sessions with on-call internists and pediatricians. The on-call doctors continue to turn in their call slips and see very ill patients during off hours. At the end of nursing coverage, incoming calls are referred directly to the physicians.

The original tele-nurse continues this work part time and is now working as an educational coordinator part time. She is formalizing the nurse's telephone role. She was instrumental in developing the call slips, standing orders, and ways of passing on information. She and the nursing coordinator of triage developed guidelines with a series of questions which telephone operators, expeditors, and unit secretaries ask patients. She has demonstrated the patient situations that can be handled over the phone and is now sharing her knowledge with the staff.

The emerging telephone training program will be given to (a) members via membership orientation programs; (b) operators, receptionists, and expeditors who answer the telephone; and (c) nurses and physicians who provide health care by telephone. This will continue to be developed through inservice education programs for small groups. Helpful literature and teaching aids are available through the various telephone companies. The final telephone training program will include a set of behavioral objectives, a pre-test, and a post-test. Currently, it is an integral part of the nursing department's orientation program.

ADVANTAGES AND DISADVANTAGES

The telephone saves time and money for both the patient and the health care agency. Unnecessary visits can be avoided and necessary visits appropriately scheduled.

Health care is more accessible when patients know a telephone system for care exists. Inaccessibility is one of the most frequent complaints about health care today. Patients do not know how to get inside the doors of today's complex medical center and often must wait weeks for an appointment even when in discomfort. With telephone service nurses solve this problem by arranging a visit and at the same time providing interim advice, a personal contact, and a sense of responsiveness. At the Harvard Community Health Plan personal contact is reinforced for each nurse identifies herself by name, and gives the patient a specific person to request on further telephone or personal contact. Accessibility offers a good deal of assurance to patients and cuts down fears and late night phone calls.

When patients know they will speak to a nurse they call with questions that they might not ask otherwise—how to prevent contracting a co-worker's hepatitis, what are the symptoms of syphilis, how many aspirin will control a temperature. Some patients who would be embarrased by asking a "stupid" or personal question appreciate the anonymity of the telephone.

Our expediter system allows the nurse to know beforehand the patient's age, sex, and problem to be dealt with. Potential aids are available—standing orders, reference books, and that unique aspect of a group practice, instant consultation. Patient information can be obtained in advance through the computerized data retrieval system, or complete records can be obtained prior to calling back. If the problem still appears insoluble during conversation, the nurse can take advantage of the hold button to work on the solution.

The use of the hold button and the time lapse in returning many calls can be either good or bad. The angry patient or a manipulative hysterical patient can benefit from a time lapse. The patient who inadequately reported symptoms or left the telephone from which he called can unfortunately be left unattended. Some patients are poor at verbal expression or are uncomfortable talking on the telephone.

ADAPTING

The most obvious disadvantage is that some people do not have telephones, especially members who are enrolled through Medicaid, Aid to Dependent Children, and such. A call from a telephone booth is often less than adequate.

The major disadvantage of giving health care by telephone is the inability to see the patient, his appearance, and his visual reaction. Interviewing skills must be sharp and somewhat different since the physical communication is absent. After a short time, nurses become sensitive to what is and is not being said.

Success of delivering nursing care by telephone is judged through the records by the confirmation of diagnosis on physical examination, resolution of a problem through follow-up conversations and, informally, by the patients themselves. After helping Ms. B. through three weeks of low-back pain, leading her from bedrest to the bathroom to how to get into a car properly, a nurse one day was greeted by a surprise visitor with an African violet in hand. "I'm Ms. B. I just had to see what your face looks like and say 'thank you'."

The plan serves primarily a young working population. This urban membership is accustomed to talking to machines and is young enough to adapt to a new system of health care. Older patients sometimes are less able to adapt or become confused more easily, and patients with a language barrier must be asked to come in even if the medical situation itself does not warrant a physical visit.

Many patients make their first contact with the nurse by telephone when they are ill and consequently under stress. This makes their adaptation to the system delicate to handle and requires continued education for both the provider and member.

Just as some patients make inadequate use of the telephone, all nurses are not ideally suited to it either. Good related clinical experience, self-confidence, sharp interviewing skills, and a good telephone voice increase the nurse's success on the telephone.

Nurses already do use the phone in this manner in various fields. It is time to go one step further, enlist the aid of the telephone company, establish goals, guidelines, and a system of evaluation, and make the most of those situations in which a patient's care can be managed via the telephone.

Section VI   Expanding the Nurse's Role in Community Health Care Delivery

Additional education and practice enabled the nurses described in these articles to expand their practices and augment the delivery of health care to persons in the community. These nurses practice in a variety of settings in the specialty roles for which they have prepared.

From the American Journal of Nursing 75:267-271, Feb. 1975. Copyright © 1975. AJN Co.

Primary Care by a Nurse Practitioner in a Rural Clinic

ROBERT OSEASOHN • MARTHA SCHWEBACK
BETTY EBERLE • RICHARD A. REID

Evaluation of services was built in when the University of New Mexico sponsored a system of health care for a small town with no physician. Primary care is provided by a nurse with telephone linkage to physicians at the university, who supervise the medical components of her care.

Several years ago, University of New Mexico staff, in collaboration with a group of local citizens, devised a system of health care for Estancia, a rural community with no physicians and little likelihood of getting one(1, 2). The basic aim was to try an approach that was new at the time —the year was 1968—having a nurse practitioner (NP) function locally, in communication for medical supervision with physicians at an urban medical center 60 miles away.

The university discussed with the staff citizens' group the nature and scope of the services that would be required. On the recommendation of the local group, a staff nurse from a large general hospital, who was the wife of a local farmer, was employed. Her past experience was varied; she had worked as a school nurse, office nurse, and in hospitals on obstetric, surgical, and emergency wards.

Preparation of the nurse began with a review of the tasks she would be expected to perform—health checkups for all ages, birth control services, antepartal and postpartal care, maintenance of the chronically ill including adjustment in medications based on observations and such indexes as blood pressure or urine testing, and care in the case of acute illness or accident. When needs could not be met locally, patients were referred to for secondary or tertiary care to the urban medical center.

The next step was to consider what additional information and skills the nurse would need in order to collect the historical data, distinguish between normal and abnormal physical findings, keep clinical records, and communicate medical data to supervisory physicians. Little attention was given to decision-making on medical conditions, as findings would dictate whether the NP would act according to written instructions or telephone for oral orders. It is important to recall that in 1968, when the system was devised, neither the supervisory physicians nor the NP had ever worked in the type of system proposed and that New Mexico law reserved diagnosis and treatment to the practice of medicine.

The training interval was six months. The community had been without locally available medical care and wanted to get started as soon as possible. Certain tasks such as performing blood counts or processing roentgenograms had been part of the NP's previous regular duties as an office nurse and she did not have to learn them from the beginning.

Before the program began, medical and nursing colleagues had to be familiarized with the proposal and its training implications so they could define their teaching roles and fit a series of exercises together into a total curriculum. Also, a final interval was reserved for observation of the NP's performance before the proposed system actually began to function.

Preparation of the NP included a review of anatomy and physiology; data collection methods—instruction in interviewing techniques, details of history and physical examination; and supervised practice. General interviewing techniques were taught by a psychiatric nurse with prior

DR. OSEASOHN *(M.D., Downstate Medical Center, University of New York, Brooklyn, N.Y.) formerly at the University of New Mexico, is professor and chairman, Department of Epidemiology and Health, McGill University, Montreal, Canada.* DR. EBERLE *(Ph.D., Case Western Reserve University, Cleveland, Ohio) is associate professor, Department of Family and Community Medicine, School of Medicine, University of New Mexico, Albuquerque.* MS. SCHWEBACK *(Alumnae-Dominician School of Nursing, Great Bend, Kan.) is the nurse practitioner whose work is described here. She continues as administrator and family nurse practitioner in the Hope Medical Center, Estancia, New Mex., which is affiliated with Presbyterian Hospital, St. Joseph Hospital, and Cooperative Health Services, Albuquerque. She lectures in the Department of Epidemiology and Community Medicine at the University of New Mexico.* DR. REID *(Ph.D., Ohio State University, Columbus) is assistant professor in the School of Business and Administrative Sciences and the Department of Family and Community Medicine, University of New Mexico.*

The study was supported in part by the Sears Roebuck Foundation, the New Mexico Regional Medical Program, and contract HSM 110-69-241, Health Services and Mental Health Administration, U.S. Department of HEW.

public health experience. Instruction in physical diagnosis was given by a group of pediatricians and internists in one-to-one tutorials with illustrative patients.

Specialty physicians and nurses dealt with specific content areas. Pediatricians discussed the approach to selected common childhood problems. Internists dealt with commonly encountered complaints among adults. A community psychiatric worker dealt with the questions posed by patients who are acutely upset, threatening suicide, depressed, or whose persistent visits are related to underlying emotional disorders.

For obstetrical and gynecological conditions, an obstetrician and nurse-midwife outlined problems concerning the premarital examination, family planning, diagnosis of pregnancy, antepartal care, emergency conduct of labor and delivery, postpartal care, periodic examinations in healthy women, and a few commonly anticipated complaints such as bleeding and discharge. Specific skills were taught, such as performance of pelvic examination and collection of material for vaginal cytology. A surgeon reviewed common emergency situations necessitating immediate referral to the urban medical center. Wound management was stressed, and indications for suturing, details of the suturing, and principles of aftercare were taught.

As the training program evolved, a record system was designed to facilitate patient care and to permit subsequent assessment of the system of care itself. A modified problem-oriented record was devised. For each patient visit, the NP was to prepare an up-to-date problem summary which showed, for each problem identified, what diagnostic and therapeutic actions were taken and the plan made for follow-up. In addition, forms were provided for details of history, physical examination, and procedures.

To test the NP's skill in physical diagnosis at the end of five months, she examined patients in the clinics of the university medical center and reported her findings by phone to supervisory physicians, who then examined the patients. When findings differed, patients were questioned or examined again. This test process was not quantitiated. However, the supervisory physician group thought her performance compared favorably with that of satisfactory interns. At that point, the rural clinic was opened.

However, training did not stop. Continuing education was built into program operation, one half-day each week.

CLINIC OPERATION

Initially, the clinic was to be staffed by two persons, the NP and a laboratory aide-receptionist.

The laboratory aide-receptionist was to handle laboratory procedures, serve as office receptionist, collect household and insurance data from new families, escort patients into examing rooms, and prepare them for examination by the NP. As the volume of clerical tasks grew, early within the first year, a clerk was hired. Part-time personnel included a housekeeper, gardener, and maintenance man. An administrative assistant at the university medical center handled details of payroll, purchasing, accounting, and personnel. When patients had to be admitted or when laboratory samples or roentgenograms were sent in, the administrative assistant expedited their processing.

Physicians supervised the medical care by written instruction and telephone. Internists handled problems of patients 15 years of age or older, and pediatricians dealt with the younger. Commonly encountered problems of infants and children could be managed with standing orders and without consulting the pediatrician. However, the NP was instructed to phone the supervisory pediatrician in defined situations or whenever doubt arose. In addition to the university-based internist and pediatrician supervisors, the NP communicated directly with physicians in the urban center when their patients sought medical help at the clinic.

The supervisory physicians usually visited the rural clinic weekly to see patients whom the NP had asked to return for examination because she could not manage their problems alone. During these visits, supervisory physicians reviewed the records of all patients who had come to the clinic during the preceding week.

The clinic was open from 8:30 A.M. until 5:00 P.M. on weekdays. Except for a brief period when a second NP was available, services were not offered at the clinic on weekends. Appointments were encouraged but not required. When appointments were not kept, clinic staff sent reminder notices by mail.

When the system was started, the community was informed that at night or on weekends they could reach urban-based physicians by calling an answering service number. However, from the outset, the answering service was rarely used and local residents called or came to the NP at her home for help. The NP was encouraged to work directly with other health and welfare personnel, school personnel, and community action groups in the county. Selected senior high school students were urged to volunteer for brief clinic assignments as part of an effort to introduce health careers to them.

EVALUATION

Task analysis. In order to learn what proportion of the NP's time was spent performing specific tasks after the clinic had been functioning for at least a year, the technique of work sampling was used. This information provided actual job descriptions and a rational basis for changing procedures.

A trained observer recorded random observations of activities of the clinic personnel. He recorded only one activity per observation. Occasionally, a staff member was performing two functions at once; for example, the NP was treating an injury and conversing with a patient. In this case, the recorded observation would be "treating the patient" since this was the primary activity. The observer was requested to make detailed notes on any particular event which seemed difficult to categorize. Only a few activities presented problems of categorization, and on review, they proved to be readily classifiable.

The NP spent about 33 percent of her time in direct contact with patients. She devoted 20 percent to record keeping and nearly that amount to telephone conversations concerning patient care. Nonproductive activities, such as idle time or meal time, consumed approximately 20 percent of her day. Comparison of findings in the present study with studies reported previously is limited due to differences in data collection methods, work-category definitions, and operational characteristics of the settings.

Nature of the care provided. Evaluation of the kind of care provided involved looking for and measuring deviations from specified standards. The first specific question we set out to answer was: are the NP's observations accurate? Accordingly, a test was conducted in which 12 infants and children who attended pediatric clinics were examined independently by the NP and a pediatrician who knew of the project, but had not participated in it.

The NP phoned her findings to one of her usual supervisory physicians. Therefore, the data compared were problems identified and related recommendations by the NP-supervisory physician linkage versus those of the practicing physician. (See table on following pages.)

Observational errors are inevitable. However, such errors must be minimized, particularly where differences may result in unfavorable outcomes to patients, that is, *when the differences make a difference.* As a rule, common sources of error are ignorance of diagnostic standards or vague standards which defy certain application. In this system, physicians have a continuing opportunity to check their findings against the NP's among patients saved for physician examination. For some chang-

Continued on p. 252

COMPARISON OF NURSE AND PEDIATRICIAN ASSESSMENT

Case No.	Nurse Practitioner (NP)— Supervisory Physician	Practicing Pediatrician (PP)	Comments
1.	Well child care (WCC) Needs rubella vaccine Rx immunize	WCC Rx none	NP's history indicated no rubella vaccine PP's history was the opposite *(Was a needed immunization omitted or an extra one given as a result of the different histories?)*
2.	WCC	WCC Strabismus	Strabismus not detected by the NP. *(Was a correctable potential "one-eyed" blindness overlooked?)*
3.	WCC Upper respiratory infection (URI) with otitis Lump at DPT site Small size, poor appetite Rx antibacterial drugs	WCC URI Lump at DPT site Rx symptomatic	PP did not consider ear drums to be abnormal. *(Were antibacterial drugs used appropriately or not?)*
4.	WCC Probably lower respiratory tract infection and otitis History of anemia Rx antibacterial drugs	WCC URI Rx symptomatic	History of previous clinic visit with penicillin treatment obtained by NP and not by the PP. She reported chest wheezes and abnormal ear drums which the PP did not. *(Again, were antibacterial drugs used appropriately or not?)*
5.	Belly pain URI, sinusitis	Belly pain	A history of frontal headaches was obtained by the NP and not by the PP. *(Both referred the child to a gastroenterologist; slightly different findings with same outcome.)*
6.	Chest pain Strep contact Breast hypertrophy	URI, pharyngitis Breast hypertrophy	The NP reported a history of strep contact which the PP did not. The PP felt the URI was viral and did not obtain a throat culture (TC). *(Again, was medication appropriate?)*

Case No.	Nurse Practitioner (NP)— Supervisory Physician	Practicing Pediatrician (PP)	Comments
7.	Viral syndrome WCC	Viral syndrome WCC	Judged pale by the PP and Hct suggested though not obtained. *(No difference in what was actually done.)*
8.	URI with otitis WCC Rx antibacterial drugs	URI WCC Rx none	Ear drums judged abnormal by the NP. *(Same issue as in cases 3 and 4. However this child was brought back to clinic three weeks later and another examining physician diagnosed acute otitis media.)*
9.	WCC Pharyngitis Pale child Rx antibacterial drugs	WCC Pharyngitis Rx antibacterial drugs	Considered pale by NP and a Hct which she obtained revealed an abnormally low value. *(Both the NP and PP recommended antibacterial drug therapy for pharyngitis; however she questioned pallor, obtained a Hct which was distinctly low, while the PP did not.)*
10.	WCC Pharyngitis Rx antibacterial drugs	WCC Pharyngitis Short stature Rx none	The PP commented on the short stature. However, the NP obtained a history of prior penicillin treatment which he did not. *(Again, were drugs used appropriately? The TC failed to show strep.)*

11.	WCC
	Possible retardation
	
	Ill child: pale,
	    purpura, stiff neck
	Cyst in neck
		WCC
		Feeding problem
		Herpes stomatitis
		Soft tissue
		    neck swelling
		Vulvo-vaginitis
			The NP thought the child more sick than the PP; she advised hospitalization. *(The child was hospitalized and did not have meningitis which concerned the NP. Later, an infected cystic hygroma was identified and treated.)*

12.	Tight foreskin Dysuria	Tight foreskin Dysuria	Agreement on problem(s) but difference as to recommendation: NP wished to refer for circumcision and the PP did not.

ing processes or unrecognized problems never saved for physicians, this method of reconciliation is obviously of limited value.

Any comparison of NP and physician findings was *bound* to reveal differences. Such differences are often a function of the clinical method itself, which is ill defined. The question remains whether a supervisory physician can depend on what the NP tells him as a basis for his further action without seeing the patient. An operational approach is suggested: keep a record concerning all patients saved for physician visits, which includes the NP's and the physician's opinion on the nature of the suspected problem or abnormal findings. Where differences occur, their basis can be sought on the spot, and explicit criteria and how to apply them defined to avoid future differences. Thus, over a period of time, one could estimate the frequency of agreement, disagreement, presumed causes for disagreement, and outcomes, where the latter might prove useful.

The second question examined dealt with the NP's ability to carry out physicians' telephone instructions. This ability had to be documented and could not be assumed, since the nurse, working in a facility over 60 miles away from the urban center, observed and managed approximately 90 percent of the patients herself. The clinic record procedure required the NP to list on the chart summary form what she did, whether she sought a telephone consultation, and with whom. When she called supervisory physicians they prepared records of the calls indicating needed actions and these memoranda were filed in patients' charts. Therefore, it was possible to review patient records and compare actions requested with actions taken. Other entries in the charts served to support whether actions had, in fact, been taken. For example, if the physician ordered a hematocrit and the NP listed the test to be done, she might also enter the result or a time of a new appointment for the test.

SAMPLE RECORDS

A sample of records of patients who visited the clinic during a five-month interval showed that the nurse took 571 of 606 actions which physicians specifically requested. She took occasional actions, which appeared to have been unauthorized, so far as could be determined from record review. The most frequent example was advice in areas where protocol called for physician consultation. In each instance, the particular advice appeared appropriate. Accordingly, evaluators concluded that the NP carried out instructions in nearly all instances (94 percent) and that discrepancies noted may have been in the clinical data recording and abstracting procedures.

There was a concern at the outset about the NP's ability to work with extramural medical colleagues and health agencies. The NP demonstrated her ability to do this successfully in a number of ways, such as arranging meetings with local school staff, welfare workers, and public health nurses to discuss problems in families for whom responsibilities were shared. Also, practicing physicians in the urban center invited her to review difficult clinical situations and spend time with them in their offices or affiliated hospitals.

The NP was instructed to place highest priority on immediate patient demands or urgent medical conditions. Details of complete history, physical examination, and laboratory procedures not directly related to the current episode could be deferred until subsequent visits. However, she was to encourage patients who sought services for acute illnesses or accidents to return for complete examinations.

Another standard of performance tested was the number of times complete histories and certain routinely recommended laboratory determinations were obtained from a group of 161 patients who sought care at the clinic at least once during a three-month interval.

Patient records revealed that the NP took complete histories of 28 percent of these patients, did purified protein derivative (PPD) skin tests or chest reontgenograms for 30 percent; ECGs for 13 percent; urinalyses for 36 percent; hematocrits for 25 percent; and cervical smears for 26 percent of the women. Histories and laboratory tests were more frequent in frequent clinic users and in older rather than younger adults.

The frequency of missed appointments in this group of 161 patients was studied, since the bulk of satisfied patients would be expected to return when asked to do so. Nearly half the patients were asked to return at least once, and the proportions increased with advancing age. Thirty-seven percent of persons asked to return did not keep their appointments. Nor did they use the clinic again during the remainder of the calendar year in which they had been seen earlier.

The records of these 161 patients were also studied to learn if potentially serious problems which the nurse might have identified were subsequently overlooked, such as finding a breast lump or blood in a stool sample and failing to take further action. Two such instances were found on review of the 161 charts. However, inquiry showed that the nurse had taken the necessary steps and that the two charts were incomplete.

In this protocol of care, it was equally important to find out what happened following visits. Accordingly, patients were urged to phone and report how they were feeling after a defined interval, even if they were much improved and needed no additional clinic visits. Supervisory physicians established this as a safety check and as a learning device for the NP. Certainly, many busy practitioners would consider such a requirement a needless burden, provided patients were improving. Accordingly, the 161 patient records were examined to learn whether outcomes had been noted. The NP had described findings at follow-up visits or telephone reports in two thirds of the records.

During the study interval, we conducted household surveys in the community to learn what factors might be associated with use and non-use of the system. One particular group of residents was identified who used the clinic once or twice and vowed never to return. Compared to the total sample, they tended to be more mobile, to report more chronic illness and related disability, to have used a wider variety of medical providers, to feel uncomfortable in a doctor-patient encounter, and to state a preference for a male physician.

Generally accepted standards are not available for ambulatory care performance, irrespective of what sort of system provides it(3). The goals of ambulatory care would appear to be problem identification; appropriate primary level diagnostic, therapeutic, and preventive action; and suitable referral or follow-up—all directed toward a favorable outcome for the patient. To attain those goals, the system of care described in this report included problem-oriented records and periodic audit. Despite the limitations in the methods employed, the steps necessary to insure favorable outcomes appear to have been taken in most instances.

REFERENCES

1. OSEASOHN, R., AND OTHERS. Rural medical care: physician's assistant linked to an urban medical center. *JAMA* 218:1417-1419, Nov. 1971.
2. OSEASOHN, R., AND SCHWEBACK, M. K. Patient care in an experimental delivery system. A case system. In *Intermediate-Level Health Practitioners*, ed. by V. W. Lippard and E. F. Purcell. New York, Josiah Macy, Jr. Foundation, 1973, pp. 198-207.
3. MCWHINNEY, I. R. Medical audit in North America. *Br. Med. J.* 2:277-279, Apr. 29, 1972.

From *Nursing Outlook* 23:381-384, June 1975. Copyright © 1975. AJN Co.

The School Nurse Practitioner

JUDITH BELLAIRE IGOE

These specially prepared nurses do comprehensive physical and psychosocial evaluations, manage a variety of minor illnesses, and place particular emphasis on teaching students to be responsible for their own health.

Seven million of the more than fifty-five million school-age children in the United States have never visited a doctor's office, clinic, or hospital except in cases of extreme illness or emergency. Millions more have emotional disturbances, perceptual handicaps, speech problems and similar difficulties for which good professional care is readily available, yet these children have never gone to where such care is administered.

Most of them, however, do go to school. The school nurse practitioner (SNP) program at the University of Colorado School of Nursing was developed to assure that schools, especially in poverty areas, could serve as the principle means of bringing complete and continuing health care to these children.* The program's goal has been to train school nurses "to offer comprehensive well-child care and to identify and assess the factors that may operate to produce learning disorders, psychoeducational problems, perceptive-cognitive difficulties, and behavior problems as well as those causing physical disease.... The purpose was to extend the capabilities of the school nurse beyond the traditional role to provide broader and more intensive attention to children's needs."(1).

The program offers a four-month intensive course in primary health care. Since the first class entered in 1970, all participants have been

---

*Initially (1970), the program was jointly sponsored by the University of Colorado Schools of Medicine and Nursing and the Denver public schools. In the fall of 1974, the University of Colorado School of Nursing assumed full responsibility for the school nurse practitioner program, incorporating it into the primary care nurse practitioner program. This large continuing education program provides a common core curriculum of primary health care skills and knowledges for nurses from a variety of fields—industry, schools, physicians' offices—as well as training in their particular specialty.

nurses already practicing in schools or other nontraditional health facilities such as juvenile detention centers, with priority given to applicants serving in disadvantaged areas. After completing the course, SNPs are required to continue their training on the job with regular consultation available from a local physician.

ROUTINE SNP ACTIVITIES

Letters, conversations, and reports from the program's sixty graduates make it possible to draw up an SNP job description based on both what SNPs are prepared to do and what they actually are doing. In general, the reports are very encouraging; the SNP does indeed do more than carry out such traditional activities as looking down throats, taking blood pressures, sending pupils home, and doing paperwork. A study made in the Denver public schools in 1972 by McAtee and Hilmar indicated that, compared with regular school nurses in the school system, the SNPs

1. tended to be more sharply focused and specific in their management of pupils' health problems;

2. excluded only about half as many pupils from school;

3. referred only about half as many pupils for consultations, care, or further evaluation, because their own management plans resolved the problems; and

4. were more likely to provide specific advice to parents, resulting in more frequent compliance with the SNP's recommendations(2).

As might be expected, in order to allow time for the diagnosis and treatment of physical and psycho-emotional ills as well as to carry out a program of health education, the SNP's daily procedure differs from that of conventional school nurses. Effective use of an SNP's time in any given school depends to a large extent on the realization by school officials that the "open door" policy of sending all complaining students to the nurse must be a thing of the past. Except in emergency situations, children who are ill are generally seen by the SNP during one of the two or three "sick periods" scheduled throughout the day. Surprisingly, SNPs

MS. IGOE (B.S.N., University of Iowa; M.S. University of Minnesota School of public Health) completed the University of Colorado pediatric nurse practitioner program in 1967 and has taught and practiced as a PNP since that time. She is now assistant professor in the University of Colorado's primary care nurse practitioner program, with special responsibilities for school nurse practitioner preparation.

report that this arrangement has been well accepted by school personnel, including principals.

PHYSICAL EXAMS

Routine examinations of well children who have been identified as non-users of traditional health facilities are handled on an appointment basis; the evaluations are similar to those performed by a private physician. A health history is taken, using a problem-oriented system of recording; this is followed by a total physical examination that includes inspection, palpation, percussion, and auscultation, with the aid of such tools as the stethoscope, otoscope, tuning fork, and sphygmomanometer. A neurological evaluation according to Vazuka's technique is also part of the examination, as is a systematic assessment of the child's psychosocial, cognitive, and perceptual development. The evaluation takes approximately forty-five minutes to one hour.

Parents of elementary school children are urged to be present at the routine exams to provide moral support for the child and pertinent data about his past and present health. Of course, results of the evaluation and recommendations for future care are shared with the parents during that same appointment.

Interestingly, SNPs are reporting that the reaction of parents is most satisfactory. Those who previously resisted any suggestion that they take their children to a traditional health care facility for preventive care are now not only letting their children be examined at school but are coming to those appointments themselves.

TREATMENT PROCEDURES

All SNPs collaborate closely with local physicians. When the SNP is new to the job, a physician is assigned to her school one half-day per week, with phone consultation readily available. During these weekly sessions, the physician and SNP jointly re-evaluate children with questionable findings, and definite decisions are reached. In addition to assisting with evaluations of students, the supervising physician also contributes informal instruction on subjects about which the SNP may still feel uncertain.

After a period of at least four months, the time spent by the physician consultant in providing medical back-up is reduced to about one half-day every other week. By this time, generally, the SNP has markedly increased her consultation with other physicians in the community.

A variety of laboratory procedures may also be part of the health evaluation. SNPs have done, for example, throat and urine cultures, hematocrits, urinalyses, sickle cell anemia screenings, pregnancy tests, and analyses of stool specimens for blood, ova, and parasites.

Once the extent and type of health care plan needed for a given child has been determined, the SNP carries it out in consultation with the physician(s) providing medical back-up. Although practices vary among school districts according to the wishes of parents and school administrators and the advice of the health professionals in the community, SNPs perform many of the following activities:

- Management of anemia due to iron deficiency with dietary instruction and therapeutic doses of ferrous sulfate.
- Management of constipation with dietary measures and, if necessary, prescription of a mild proprietary laxative.
- Management of minor allergic conditions such as allergic rhinitis with proprietary antihistaminic medications.
- Management of dermatological conditions such as tinea capitis, seborrhea, tinea corporis, pediculosis, ichthyosis, impetigo, atopic dermatitis, and insect bites, with appropriate medications.
- Management of minor upper respiratory conditions including dispensing such proprietary drugs as analgesics, antipyretics, cough remedies, and nose drops.
- Management of bacterial infections—for example, beta hemolytic strep throat infections. This usually involves notifying parents of the results of throat cultures and recommending medical treatment in a traditional health care facility. In those rare instances where it is known that the child has had previous similar infections with no follow-up treatment and parents continue to refuse to seek treatment, the SNP and her medical colleague may decide to provide antibiotic therapy in school.
- Management of trauma and injury with emergency first-aid measures.

PSYCHOSOCIAL EVALUATION

The SNP's evaluation is designed to yield specific information about a student's psychosocial health status, as well as his physical condition. This information is gathered through observation as well as verbal and nonverbal communication. A variety of psychological data collection tools are also used.

Just as care plans for physical ills are often formulated and carried out by the SNP in cooperation with a physician, in the case of emotional difficulties (e.g., school phobia, immaturity, poor self-image), consultants with expertise in this area are also employed. The SNP may choose to refer the student immediately to other school or community professionals such as physicians, psychiatrists, psychologists, counselors, or social workers; she may decide to institute her own management plan for a while, postponing evaluation by others to a later date; or she may decide that a joint management plan is warranted and make arrangements with other professionals to insure that all phases of the plan are developed and implemented simultaneously.

In both the planning and follow-up stages, SNPs also consult a variety of other professionals, including classroom teachers, school administrators, speech therapists, and public health nurses. All of these have been most helpful in providing both historical background on students and suggestions for their psychosocial care.

At present, the management plans most often used by SNPs in dealing with emotional problems involve behavior modification techniques, usually developed and implemented in collaboration with consulting psychologists. Thus, pupils with behavior problems seen in the school clinic on a follow-up basis are handled according to a carefully planned routine. This directed intervention certainly seems to be more successful than the old custom of a friendly but ill-defined chat with the school nurse.

Naturally, all pupils whose health evaluations result in the development of a care plan are closely followed. Detailed reports of the initial work-up and subsequent visits enable SNPs to continue to evaluate the child's progress and to modify the care plan if necessary.

SNPs with secretarial assistance find that they spend less time than previously in the actual preparation of these work-ups and progress reports. Since most school nurses cannot take on the extra duties associated with becoming an SNP unless they are relieved of some routine tasks, school health aides—both adults and high school students—must be available to assist with routine clerical and minor first-aid activities.

HEALTH EDUCATION ACTIVITIES

In many facilities, the most efficient and least utilized health care service is health education. Working in the schools, SNPs are able to concentrate on this very effective form of prevention in a variety of ways. Some use traditional methods, such as one-to-one discussions with students during appointments or sick call periods, classroom presentations and discussions, and consultation with teachers. However, many SNPs say that the health education seminars included in their nurse practitioner course influenced them to broaden their approach to include two additional functions: 1) to increase pupils' ability to assume greater responsibility and independence with respect to their own health care; and 2) to enable pupils to develop confidence in their right to expect that a collaborative, rather than subservient, relationship can exist between themselves and health professionals.

SNPs report that in order to achieve the first goal, students must be presented with material that they can actually apply to their daily lives. This is best done when the pupil receives some specific, self-satisfying responsibility for his own health care on a regular basis in conjunction with the health education program. Specifically, SNPs have extended health education beyond the routine skills of hand-washing, toothbrushing, and minor first aid to more complex practices such as maintaining one's own immunization records; at some schools this is introduced in the fourth grade

The scientific rationale for immunizations is always taught before the actual responsibility for the records is delegated, so that pupils have a rational foundation for the decisions they are beginning to make about their own health care. In fact, SNPs report that many students now call it to their parents' attention when booster injections and additional immunizations are required.

EVALUATION CRITERIA

Another example of this participatory approach to health education involves teaching fifth and sixth graders some specific criteria for evaluation of the severity of such symptoms as headache and abdominal pains, in order that they may themselves decide whether further evaluation by a nurse or physician is needed. Observation and follow-up indicate that the students make rational judgments as to what to do and that they are eager to assume the responsibility involved.

Finally, SNPs are teaching junior and senior high school students how to assume greater responsibility for the self-management of minor illnesses and symptoms.

The second goal—to help pupils develop a collaborative relationship between themselves and health professionals—was felt to be especially important, since such relationships lead consumers to be open in expressing opinions to health professionals, resulting in more effective and mutually acceptable solutions to health problems. This contrasts with the submissive-authoritarian relationship which is still evident today between health consumers and professionals and which, unfortunately, often results in consumer resistance to the health professional's treatment plan(3).

With SNP guidance, pupils learn what to expect from health personnel when they visit a health facility and what their own responsibilities are during such a visit. For instance, the contents of a health history are specifically explained by the SNP; then, once students understand the reasons for certain questions (e.g., family history) they are taught to compile their own health histories. This learning can be immediately (and satisfyingly) applied when the pupil shares his health history and other information with health professionals in settings other than the school clinic.

PATTERNS OF SNP PRACTICE

Information gleaned from graduates of our SNP program indicate three general patterns of SNP practice.

The first and most common pattern is for the SNP to assume responsibility for the total school health program for approximately 1,400 children, with the assistance of an aide who takes care of most of the clerical work, schedules appointments, and triages simple conditions in which he or she has been instructed. This recommended ratio was established after SNP graduates reported that, in general, 25 percent of their total school populations failed to utilize traditional health care facilities except in times of emergency. It is therefore estimated that an SNP could satisfactorily accommodate approximately 300 pupils per year in her program of health evaluation, education, and management while administering the overall health program for her school.

Nurses who function in this pattern of practice also provide improved evaluative services to any child who complains of illness or injury. In those instances where the child has a regular source of health care outside the school clinic, the SNP prepares a specific written referral of her evaluation.

The second pattern of practice is for the SNP to visit a number of schools to evaluate only those children in need of a comprehensive health appraisal. In these situations, follow-up services are provided by the regular school nurse or ancillary personnel, who are also responsible for the overall school health program.

The third and least common pattern involves assigning the SNP to the diagnostic screening clinic operated by the school district. In the limited instances where this has occurred, SNPs are most frequently involved in individual health evaluations of children experiencing learning difficulties rather than in the delivery of ongoing comprehensive health care.

SUMMARY

Whatever the specific details of their practices, SNPs have shown themselves able to function effectively in their expanded roles because they have assumed more responsibility, initiative, interdependence, and independence in caring for children. Specifically, they have learned to be confident of their decision-making abilities, to adapt themselves to an expanded framework of nursing, and to regard themselves as highly qualified professionals.

What this means to the individual nurse practitioner, the parent, and—most important—the child is well summed up in these remarks from Larea Younkman, SNP in the Denver Public Schools: "Previously," she writes, "my recommendations to the parents as to what to do and when, such as seeking medical attention, were frequently too general and consequently not heeded by the parent. Now when I talk to a parent, I am not only confident of my findings but I'm also much more convinced that what I suggest is necessary. As a result, parents are looking at SNPs differently, trusting our judgment, and, I think, following through on the advice we offer to a greater extent than previously."

Thus the SNP could well be the vital bridge between this country's traditional system of health care delivery and those children who are deprived of the care they need through reluctance, ignorance, parental apathy, or lack of available health care facilities.

REFERENCES

1. SILVER, H. K. The school nurse practitioner program; a new and expanded role for the school nurse. *JAMA* 216:1332-1334, May 24, 1971.
2. HILMAR, N. A. AND MCATEE, P. A. The school nurse practitioner and her practice; a study of traditional and expanded health care responsibilities for nurses in elementary schools. *J. Sch. Health* 43:431-441, Sept. 1973.
3. KALISCH, B. J. Of half gods, half mortals: Aesculapian authority. *Nurs. Outlook* 23:22-28, Jan. 1975.

From *Nursing Outlook* 23:369-373, June 1975. Copyright © 1975. AJN Co.

Expanding the Public Health Nurse's Role in Child Care

MARGARET O'BRIEN • MARGERY MANLY
MARGARET C. HEAGARTY

The problems and adjustments in preparing staff nurses as pediatric nurse associates in one urban health department are discussed as well as the ways these nurses improved services to parents and children.

"The entire staff were both pleased and gratified with the smiles and appreciation of the mother of an eight-month-old boy. He was first seen by the pediatric nurse associate (PNA) at six weeks of age and was admired by the staff. He was a cheerful infant, very active, and sociable. Because of financial distress, the mother had to go to work when the child when six months old. The boy was left with a baby sitter and saw the mother about two hours a day. Two months later, the mother brought him to the clinic because he had a cold. He had gained only two ounces, was less active, apathetic, whining, and had lost his appetite. No physical defects were noted. During the week, he was seen three times by the doctor and the PNA, and the cause of his condition was determined— maternal deprivation.

"The PNA held conferences with the mother to explain the cause of the baby's ailment and discuss ways of dealing with it. The mother continued to work but was able to adjust her hours so that she could keep the baby at home during the day. Within a short time, the baby gained weight, his appetite improved, and he became more active. The mother is pleased and appreciative of the guidance and support given to her by the staff and especially the PNA."

This little anecdote is typical of reports coming into the Bureau of

Public Health Nursing about the activities of the new pediatric nurse associates now working in the child health stations of the Department of Health of the City of New York.

Who are these new nursing professionals? How did this innovation in nursing begin and why?

In the early 1970s, the administrative staff—both medical and nursing—within the health department became concerned about the rising infant mortality and morbidity rates in our city. For instance, in the first six months of 1971, the infant mortality rate per 1,000 live births in this country was 19.4; in New York City, the rate was 21 per 1,000. However, in many districts of the city, the rate was even higher—32.4 per 1,000 in one area and 26.9 in another.

WELL-CHILD CARE VISITS

At that time, the department operated 87 child health stations throughout the city, the largest such network in the nation. These clinics accounted for 377,092 well-child care visits involving about 160,000 infants and preschool children. In a city our size, these figures represent only a small fraction of the total child care needs. These health stations were staffed by physicians, public health nurses, public health assistants, and some clerks.

With an infant mortality rate higher than the national average and with limited physician manpower, the department sought alternative measures to improve its child care program. Around the nation, pediatric nurse associate programs, as first described by Silver, were developing as a means of expanding the nursing role and of improving the quality and quantity of child care.* We believed that if our staff public health nurses were given a similar learning program, they would be prepared to provide greater depth and skill in delivering child care.

PRESENT PRACTICES

Traditionally, public health nurses in the department have been responsible for such activities as casefinding and referral to community agencies. In addition, each nurse carries a selected caseload of families with special medical and social problems. They appraise existing or potential health needs of individuals and families and interpret to patients the implications of the diagnosis and the nature of treatment recommended by physicians. Primarily, the public health nurse does family-centered nursing by assisting the individual and the family with

---

*Silver, H. K. and others. A program to increase health care for children; the pediatric nurse practitioner program. *Pediatrics* 39:756-760, May 1967.

problems—medical, social, or economic—that interfere with the family's ability to cope with the activities of daily living.

We wanted to build on these nurses' experience and expertise and extend their skills to include doing physical examinations and giving treatment for the minor illnesses of childhood. In other words, we wished to prepare them to assume responsibility for that portion of the physician's role that could safely and adequately be handled by a public health nurse who had received additional educational preparation. She would then be able to assume total responsibility for the child and the family, providing both the medical and the public health nursing components of care.

PROGRAM TO EXPAND ROLE

With this goal in mind, exploratory meetings were held between staff of the health department and faculty, both nursing and medical, at Cornell University Medical Center, the result of which was agreement by the medical center's faculty to conduct an educational program to prepare public health nurses employed by the department for this new role. This was the beginning of what has evolved into a unique experiment in collaboration between a large and busy health department and an equally large and complex university medical center.

As work on the pediatric nurse associate curriculum began, the members of the university faculty—both physicians and nurses—worked with their counterparts in the health department to ensure not only that the educational goals for the program were attained, but also that the needs of the health department and the future roles of the students were considered. To accomplish this goal, an experienced supervising public health nurse from the department was assigned to the university faculty to interpret the needs and procedures of the department.

The program that evolved followed closely the guidelines established by the American Nurses' Association and the American Academy of

MS. O'BRIEN (Misericordia Hospital School of Nursing, New York; M.S., St. John's University, New York; M.P.H., Columbia University) is director, Bureau of Public Health Nursing, Department of Health, City of New York. MS. MANLY (St. John's Hospital School of Nursing, New York; M.A., Teachers College, Columbia University) is a supervising public health nurse in the Department of Health and an instructor in the Cornell University programs described here. DR. HEAGARTY (M.D., University of Pennsylvania, Philadelphia) is an associate professor of pediatrics and director, Division of Pediatric Ambulatory Care, New York Hospital-Cornell Medical Center, New York.

Pediatrics for the preparation of pediatric nurse associates in an expanded role in any setting—clinics, private physicians' offices, or in independent practice. The course was of one year's duration. The first four months consisted of intensive didactic and practical experiences, and the following eight months were spent in a closely supervised internship within the child health stations. However, because of the background of the nurses and the fact that they all worked in one agency—the health department—certain elements were tailored to their needs. For example, a general format of recording was taught and then was adapted to the forms used in the child health stations. In addition, laboratory methods of screening for lead poisoning differed in the medical center and the health department, so both methods were taught.

At the same time, most of the nurses had strengths to build upon as well as a few deficits to be remedied. For instance, they were strong on interviewing and teaching skills, but were weak on current medications. Therefore, several classes were given to a review of pharmacology and the effects and contraindications of medications used in the health department's treatment protocols for children.

SELECTION OF CANDIDATES

The health department and the university jointly engaged in the selection of the prospective students. As with any innovation, the first step was to inform all health department staff of the new program and to invite all interested candidates to apply. The response was overwhelming: two-thirds of the nursing staff indicated interest. The director of public health nursing formed a committee composed of representatives of the administrative staff and the bargaining agency for the nursing staff to review each candidate's personnel file, including work performance and previous academic achievement. Only nurses who had worked in the department at least three years were considered.

The candidates selected were tested by the university, using the National League of Nursing prebaccalaureate examinations. On the basis of their reading comprehension and verbal ability scores, the final candidates—fifteen for the first class—were chosen during a conference between the director of nursing and the university faculty.

The health department agreed to pay the full salary of the nurses during the year of study and supervised experience. The cost to the agency, then, depends on the salary of the nurses involved, plus their fringe benefits. In addition, the department paid for the instruments (stethoscope, otoscope, et cetera) and books used by the nurses. A federal grant covered the cost to the university.

STUDENT'S CLINICAL EXPERIENCE

In the first four months of the course, most of the 63 sessions allotted to clinical experience took place in the department's child health stations in Manhattan and the South Bronx. The class of 15 students was divided into four groups. A pediatrician preceptor from the medical center was assigned to each group on a rotation basis. Every pediatrician on staff participated in the program, teaching in the classroom setting or in the clinical area. The three nursing instructors involved in the program also divided their time among the four groups.

At the child health station, each nurse would select a patient from those attending the regular clinic session. She would elicit a history, perform a complete physical examination, and record her findings. The physician preceptor would reexamine the child, affirm or correct her findings, and plan with the nurse the health supervision of the child. The physician's main function during the session was to teach the nurses in his group. The doctor would also submit a written evaluation of each student after each clinical session.

The nursing instructor would usually observe one student during the session, concentrating on history and physical techniques, interviewing skills, ability to correlate theory to practice, and written records—in general, assessing the weaknesses and strengths of the student. Findings and suggestions would be discussed with the student after each session.

During the next phase of the program, each student was again assigned to a child health station. She spent three days a week there working with a health department physician as her preceptor. One day a week was devoted to follow-up of her caseload. She would check on positive findings, visit delinquents, and arrange special conferences with parents, either at the clinic or in their homes. She also visited personnel in local community agencies to whom she referred clients. On the fifth day, she returned to Cornell for seminars, lectures, and additional clinical experience.

PROBLEMS ENCOUNTERED

During both phases of the clinical practice experience, some problems were encountered and adjustments had to be made. Space was a big factor. Each group of four PNA trainees required privacy, quiet, an area to work in, and equipment for examining their patients during the usual bustle of regular clinic sessions. The facilities were often overcrowded, and the nurse in charge frequently had to give up her space. At the same time, the head nurse had to be available to give needed information to the

PNA trainees regarding local resources.

Stress became more apparent during the internship period. The first month was a difficult time for everyone. The physician preceptor had doubts about his role and responsibilities of teaching the PNA. The time the preceptor devoted to the PNA slowed the clinic flow, and both staff and parents became impatient. The staff were bewildered about the time it took the PNA to examine a child and record her findings. In the first month, each trainee saw only one or two patients per session. The trainee was also under great strain during this period. She was in a different area, had new coworkers, missed the companionship of her group, and was very much aware of the many eyes upon her. Interestingly, the nursing staff were usually more critical of the trainees than was the doctor.

This stress can be lessened with good communications and orientation for all of the staff. The PNA began to gain satisfaction when the families visited several times and when she received confirmation regarding her findings. This became more apparent in the fifth and sixth month of internship.

ACCEPTANCE BY CO-WORKERS

One major adjustment was acceptance and recognition by co-workers of a nursing colleague in the new extended role. Generally, good rapport was established because other staff nurses were excited and delighted to see members of their profession advancing into the extended role. But, as one would expect, some of them resented the fact that they were not selected for this program and exhibited all of the symptoms of the "why her, not me" syndrome.

The preceptors in the clinics—physicians regularly assigned there— also had problems adjusting to the trainees. In addition to their duties as clinic physicians, they assumed responsibility for reviewing the physical examination and findings of the nurse and gave individual instruction related to particular findings. Some were unwilling or reluctant to assume this role. As the nursing profession moved ahead into the realm of what to many was the physician's province, doctors were threatened and concerned because "nurses are taking our jobs." However, as the internship proceeded, an excellent and mutually respectful relationship developed between the nurses and the preceptors.

OUTCOMES OF THE PROGRAM

The management of any program includes planning, implementing, and evaluating results. The latter aspect is often the most difficult and, therefore, most often neglected. Properly done, the evaluation tool should be built into the program and, more important, meticulously implemented.

Beginning with the internship, special statistical reports were submitted monthly by the interns to the director of public health nursing. These reports were reviewed and monitored for evidence of the nurse associates' progress, but on a much broader scale they provided evidence of the impact of this innovation upon the total program for child health in this city.

And there has been progress: 44 public health nurses have completed the PNA program to date. Beginning with their internship and in the following 21 months, the first group of 15 nurse associates have managed 21,779 visits to the child health stations. In 13 months, the second group of 15 nurses had a patient census of 14,783 visits. In 1973, these two groups of nurse associates, some fully trained and others partly, provided services for 6 percent of the total volume of children seen in the child health stations.

During the internship, the productivity rate of the interns increased over the 8-month period. At first, each PNA saw only one or two patients in a 3-hour session. By the completion of the internship, each one saw three to four patients in the same period. Obviously, this low productivity rate is initially costly and must be considered in the planning and implementation of a new program. The reasons for this are not only the newly developing skills of the students but also the insistence of both the university and the health department that this 8-month internship be considered an educational process. The students were closely supervised by both their physician preceptors and university faculty, thereby ensuring the quality of their educational experience at the expense of service requirements.

Another index of educational progress was comparison of the PNAs' scores from pre- and post-examinations. They took the National League of Nursing test in nursing of children on admission to the course and after completing the four month didactic part of the program. The average score on admission was 38.6 percent and, after four months, it was 82.55 percent.

PROVIDING TOTAL CHILD CARE

In the 8-month period between November 1973 and June 1974, 29 fully trained pediatric nurse associates worked within the child health stations. On average, each PNA saw 4.4 patients in each 3-hour session, as compared to a physician who saw an average of 10.8 patients per session. While the PNA gives total care to the child, including not only the physical examination but also counseling of the parent, follow-up, and any referrals necessary for the child or the family, the physician's task usually does not include these more traditional elements of public health nursing. Before our PNA program, each patient was seen by a physician as well as a public nurse, whereas the PNA combined the two aspects of care in the one visit.

Traditionally, the child health station has not been equipped to provide total care of the child—both when sick and well. Previous studies have indicated that about 25 percent of the children attending well-child stations are referred for medical follow-up. In the eight months in which 29 fully trained nurse associates worked within the system, the average referral rate ranged from 8 to 15 percent. While these figures indicate a fairly wide variation in the rate of referral among this group of nurse associates, this rate is lower than the average for the entire child health system.

In a sample of referrals made from the child health stations to another treatment agency by the PNA and her physician preceptor, 75 percent of the referred conditions were confirmed. As might be expected, such conditions included minor orthopedic defects, cardiac murmurs, and often the common respiratory illnesses of childhood. Currently, 18 of the well-child clinics have been converted to pediatric treatment centers, which diminishes the necessity for referral of these minor conditions to other pediatric resources.

The PNA working in these centers functions within guidelines developed by both the pediatricians in the department's Bureau of Child Health and the nursing administrative and consultant staff in the Bureau of Public Health Nursing. Standing orders for treatment are clearly spelled out, and the PNAs may dispense medications according to these orders. Upon graduation, the PNA assumes total responsibility for her own caseload, but consults with the physician when necessary. In addition, at least twice a month, the PNA and the physician have a conference concerning the total caseload.

When an evalutation of a program such as ours is conducted, several other considerations must be included:

- *Cost.* The pediatric nurse associate is costly during the internship period, particularly in its early months, because of the nurses' low productivity rate. As their productivity increases, their cost decreases.

- *Supervision.* To preserve the educational component, the faculty of the university must be part of the ongoing supervision of the interns. Therefore, a joint program of supervision should be planned for and provided by both the educational institution and the health department.

- *Communication.* There must be continuous dialogue between the university faculty and the health department administrative personnel to solve problems, adjust the curriculum, and insure a smooth working relationship. To help accomplish this goal, an advisory committee of health department personnel and university faculty met monthly for these purposes.

Perhaps most important, a climate of confidence must exist between the members of each agency so that mutual understanding and agreement can be reached in the development and the implementation of a worthwhile program. Obviously, at times frustration and misunderstandings occur but, with commitment and trust, problems can be solved mutually.

CONCLUSIONS

We believe that this program not only improves the quality of health care for children, but it also develops a special relationship between the parent and the PNA in which both share a common interest and concern in the welfare of the individual child. For example, a mother recently took her child south to visit relatives. While there, the child became ill, was seen by a physician, and a regimen of treatment prescribed. The mother telephoned the PNA from the south for reassurance. This is a typical example of the confidence the parents have in this nurse.

Our experience thus far has been with the preschool child. We believe another group of youngsters in our city can benefit from the ministrations of the pediatric nurse associate—the children of school age. We are assigning some of our PNAs to the school health program; however, it is too early to evaluate their contribution, but we predict they will be as successful in that setting as in the child health stations.

We believe that in expanding the role of our staff public health nurses, we are laying a foundation for future generations. The leaders and pacesetters of the future will come from this present group of children. In establishing improved health care for this age group, we are helping to insure healthy adults and citizens.

From the *American Journal of Nursing* 75:1298-1299, Aug. 1975. Copyright © 1975. AJN Co.

The Maternal-Child Nurse Practitioner

MARIE SCOTT BROWN • CAROL O'MEARA • SUSAN KROWLEY

These nurses bridge the gap between obstetric and pediatric care.

For the last two years a pilot program aimed at developing a new type of nurse practitioner has been under way at the University of Colorado. The idea grew out of eight years of experience with the Pediatric Nurse Practitioner Program and concern over a real gap in the health care of women and children.

A common experience for pediatric nurse practitioners is to become involved with a baby at his first well-child visit when he is six weeks of age. It does not take long to realize that the mother's plans for the baby, attitudes toward the baby, and decisions concerning the baby have been established long before this time. The nurse often finds she is nine months too late.

The mother also suffers from this late introduction to the nurse who will care for her child. In this country women encounter an abrupt change in health care between the time they are pregnant and the time they begin caring for their newborns. This lack of continuity is apparent in both medical and nursing care and comes at a truly crucial time in the mother-

MARIE SCOTT BROWN, *R.N., PH.D., is an assistant professor at the University of Colorado, Denver.* CAROL O'MEARA, *R.N., M.S., is a maternal-child nurse practitioner in the Neighborhood Health Program. Denver, Colorado.* SUSAN KROWLEY, *R.N., B.S.N., is a clinical nurse in maternal child care at University of California Hospital, San Diego.*

child relationship. The role of the maternal-child nurse practitioner was evolved in an attempt to bridge this gap and a program was instituted to prepare a nurse to give primary care to the woman beginning during pregnancy and continuing through her child-rearing years. Two of the authors were student participants in the pilot intensive, four-month, educational program, and now are practicing maternal-child nurse practitioners.

OUR STUDENT EXPERIENCE

A typical day in the life of a maternal-child nurse practitioner student begins at 8:00 A.M. with a two-hour lecture in physical diagnosis, followed by a practice session which might focus on checking ears, looking at tonsils, or listening to lung sounds. Later in the morning there is a lecture on various pathologies she is likely to encounter, and finally, during lunch time she sees a film depicting such things as the proper methods of palpating the abdomen and measuring fetal growth.

The afternoon is devoted to the most important part of the program—clinical practice in either ob-gyn or well-baby clinic, depending on the day. In the ob-gyn clinic, she begins seeing women under the direct observation of the obstetrician. Later she sees them alone and uses the physician only for consultation. She learns many skills including pelvic exams, insertion of IUDs, fitting of diaphragms, measuring fetal growth, Leopold maneuvers, and listening for fetal heart tones. In well-baby clinic, she practices taking a complete history and learning how to use this important tool as a basis for counseling parents. It is here that she develops a beginner's proficiency in the physical examination of the young child.

The evening schedule begins with pediatric ward rounds and then there might be an OB lecture, a neurological seminar, an experience in VD clinic, or a class in natural childbirth to attend.

One of the most interesting facets of the pilot program was the research project in which students took part. As data collectors in a project comparing the effectiveness of various methods of breast preparation for breast feeding, students instructed women prenatally in one of three methods of breast preparation and then followed each one and her breast-feeding baby for 10 days postpartum using specific objective criteria for evaluating nipple tenderness. Many questions on infant and breast feeding came up and much counseling took place during the study.

PRACTITIONER EXPERIENCE

Although graduates of this program can function in many areas (rural practice, hospital outpatient departments, public health agencies, with general practitioners, and with private group practices) two of the authors' experience has been in a prepaid health program which has both an obstetric and a pediatric clinic. Here each patient is seen initially by the nurse and then on the second visit by the physician. With his approval, the nurse then follows her exlusively until the third trimester of pregnancy. Then the woman sees the physician and nurse practitioner at alternate visits.

After an initial introduction and explanation of her role, the nurse begins the initial visit with a complete antepartal history and basic physical examination, part of which is a pelvic examination including speculum inspection, bimanual palpation, and clinical pelvimetry. The nurse obtains specimens for such screening tests as urinalysis, Pap smear, and gonoccocal cultures and orders the appropriate blood tests. Counseling the mother on nutrition, exercise, dental care, sexual activity, and danger signs is an important part of this visit and will be reviewed and discussed on future visits.

Before she leaves, the woman is given a card with "her nurse's" name and number and is encouraged to call any time she has a concern. On subsequent visits, we continue to monitor her pregnancy and counsel her on all aspects of maternal and child care.

Although the nurse does not deliver the baby, her role continues in the delivery room, where she provides physical care and emotional support for the parents. She does an immediate evaluation of the infant in the delivery room, determines gestational age, and monitors vital signs. Later, in the nursery, she performs a complete physical examination of the newborn and, with the physician, watches for signs of illness in the neonate.

During the immediate postpartum period she makes daily visits to the mother in the hospital and evaluates her physical and emotional adjustment. In the later postpartum period, the nurse sees the mother and baby in the office where she will evaluate the postpartal progress, perform physical and pelvic examinations, and advise on specific methods of family planning. She continues to provide comprehensive well child care to the baby, performing necessary evaluative procedures, including the health history, physical examination, routine screening, immunizations, and counseling.

The experience of maternal-child nurse practitioners has proven to us the tremendous value of this type of continuity of care and patients appear to appreciate its increased effectiveness.

E-89